The International Librar

CHARACTER AND THE UNCONSCIOUS

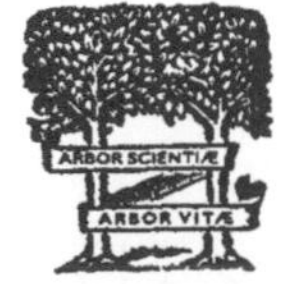

Founded by C. K. Ogden

The International Library of Psychology

PSYCHOANALYSIS
In 28 Volumes

I	The Elements of Practical Psycho-Analysis	*Bousfield*
II	A Neglected Complex and its Relation to Freudian Psychology	*Bousfield*
III	The Omnipotent Self	*Bousfield*
IV	The Social Basis of Consciousness	*Burrow*
V	What is Psychoanalysis?	*Coriat*
VI	The Psychoanalytic Theory of Neurosis	*Fenichel*
VII	The Technique of Psycho-Analysis	*Forsyth*
VIII	Leonardo da Vinci	*Freud*
IX	Totem and Taboo	*Freud*
X	Wit and its Relation to the Unconscious	*Freud*
XI	Morbid Fears and Compulsions	*Frink*
XII	Facts and Theories of Psychoanalysis	*Hendrick*
XIII	Fathers or Sons?	*Hopkins*
XIV	Neurosis and Human Growth	*Horney*
XV	The Neurotic Personality of Our Time	*Horney*
XVI	New Ways in Psychoanalysis	*Horney*
XVII	Our Inner Conflicts	*Horney*
XVIII	Self-Analysis	*Horney*
XIX	Childhood and After	*Isaacs*
XX	Social Development in Young Children	*Isaacs*
XXI	Problems in Psychopathology	*Mitchell*
XXII	The Psychoanalytic Method	*Pfister*
XXIII	The Trauma of Birth	*Rank*
XXIV	On the Bringing Up of Children	*Rickman*
XXV	Conflict and Dream	*Rivers*
XXVI	Psychoanalysis and Suggestion Therapy	*Stekel*
XXVII	Psychoanalysis and Behaviour	*Tridon*
XXVIII	Character and the Unconscious	*van der Hoop*

CHARACTER AND THE UNCONSCIOUS

A Critical Exposition of the Psychology of Freud and Jung

J H VAN DER HOOP

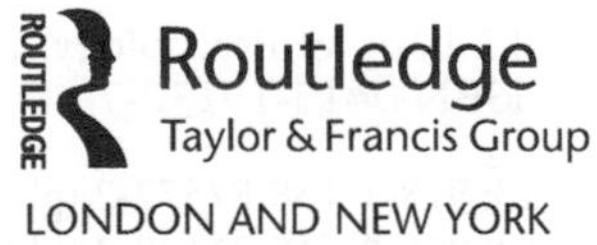

LONDON AND NEW YORK

First published in 1923 by
Routledge
2 Park Square, Milton Park, Abingdon, Oxfordshire OX14 4RN
711 Third Avenue, New York, NY 10017

First issued in paperback 2014

Routledge is an imprint of the Taylor and Francis Group, an informa business

British Library Cataloguing in Publication Data
A CIP catalogue record for this book
is available from the British Library

Character and the Unconscious
ISBN 0415-21109-3
Psychoanalysis: 28 Volumes
ISBN 0415-21132-8
The International Library of Psychology: 204 Volumes
ISBN 0415-19132-7

ISBN 13: 978-1-138-87572-2 (pbk)
ISBN 13: 978-0-415-21109-3 (hbk)

PREFACE

THIS book is intended to be a critical survey of the psychology of Freud and Jung. Although many introductions to this subject have already been published in English, little attention has so far been paid to the causes of divergence in the theories of these scientists, who originally were in complete agreement with each other. This question should be of interest to all who are not content merely to condemn and ignore the point of view which they do not approve of. I believe that only a thorough understanding of this problem will enable us to realise the significance of the new psychology, which cannot grow into a harmonious system of scientific theory unless psychologists will take the trouble to investigate the origin of existing differences of opinion.

I have tried to avoid a detailed description both of psycho-analytical technique, and of the origins of various neuroses. Those subjects seem to me too difficult and complicated, and hardly ripe enough for this kind of general treatment. It is important to realise that psycho-analysis is a most subtle and difficult method, which leads to very complicated psycho-pathological theories; otherwise we might be tempted to form premature and one-sided judgments, and there would be a danger that practitioners and others might attempt to treat patients without sufficient scientific training, and so might bring psycho-analysis into discredit.

This book is the result of nine years' intensive study of the practice and theory of psycho-analysis. It was written before the publication of Jung's *Psychological*

Types, after which I revised and added to the fifth chapter, which treats of the psychological types. Thus the book everywhere represents my own views, though I need hardly say how much they owe to both Freud and Jung.

The reader will perceive that I have represented psychology as a science that is still in a state of growth. New experiences are continually accumulating, and giving rise to new and divergent generalisations. Those who have no opportunity of judging from their own experience may easily be confused by this mass of facts and opinions, and will find it very difficult to obtain a clear survey of the whole. Notwithstanding these difficulties, I think that a somewhat general account may be of great use, because the subject-matter of this new psychology has aroused such universal interest, and is so closely connected with many contemporary problems. Our time is full of external and internal strife. In the social world we are faced by many intricate problems, whose solution requires a profound understanding of the human mind. But in our own lives too, we all of us meet with dilemmas and uncertainties which should make us eagerly welcome a science which may throw light on the hidden depths of the soul. I hope that this book may help to convince the reader that the new psychology will in time fulfil many of our expectations.

Next to Mrs R. C. Trevelyan, I wish to express my thanks to Mr R. C. Trevelyan for his revision of the translation, to Miss Constance E. Long, M.D., and to Miss Sybil I. Welsh, M.D., for their criticism of the fifth chapter.

J. H. van der HOOP.

CONTENTS

Character and the Unconscious

CHAPTER I

THE ORIGINS OF PSYCHO-ANALYSIS

ANY enquiry into the origin of psycho-analytical research inevitably leads us into the region of medical science, and more especially to the consideration of that peculiar disease, hysteria. The new psychological outlook did not arise from that psychology which has been evolved, and is still being developed, by philosophers and academic psychologists ; it has been the necessary outcome of daily medical practice. We will begin by considering the attitude of the doctor towards his patient, when he desires to determine the nature and causes of a disease. He will carefully examine all the physical symptoms, and note the presence of any peculiar phenomena from which he may infer that a particular organ is ailing. It may happen that these phenomena cannot be ascribed to any physical cause, that they originate in a hidden distress, in over-strain or inner conflict. In the old days when no proper line of demarcation was drawn between the two sets of causes, disease of any sort was attributed to mysterious forces, such as the hand of God, the workings of the devil and of evil spirits, or the malign influence of one individual upon another. There has been a gradual improvement since then ; but even to-day the origin and the cure of disease are imputed to hidden causes by the superstitious. Considerable progress was effected in medical science by the development of the natural sciences, and many fantastic theories were uprooted by more methodical and acute observation. The patient's physical condition was examined with ever increasing care; the nature of the disease was circumscribed within better defined limits, and the causes of many ailments became better known. But this advance in knowledge was restricted almost entirely to the physical world. The state of the patient's mind was overlooked, as it was thought impossible to apply here the same accurate methods of observation and experiment. To a great extent this is still the case, and many well known scientists do not believe in the possibility of dealing with psychology in a really scientific manner. Although the symptoms and the course of mental diseases have been patiently and carefully described, reviewed and classified, in practice these labours have not yielded anything like the harvest which mankind has garnered from the natural sciences. So far, we have scarcely advanced beyond the stage of superficial generalisation. Now, however, owing to our growing interest in the workings of the mind, new paths are being discovered which will lead to increasingly practical results.

There was something accidental in the origins of psychological research. During the latter half of the previous century, Charcot, then professor in Paris, achieved world-wide fame by his penetrating investigations into all manner of nerve troubles. He was able to point out that the cause of many cases of paralysis, of physical disturbance of the senses and of the muscles, was to be looked for in certain diseases of the brain and the spine. A slight inflammation or tumour somewhere in this delicate nerve tissue was sometimes found to be the explanation of all sorts of complicated symptoms. After much further enquiry into the nature of nervous diseases, Charcot dedicated himself to the study of hysterical phenomena. At that time the greatest confusion reigned on the subject. Most students preferred not to deal with it at all, and hysterical patients were often looked upon as frauds and impostors. Charcot however was compelled to be interested in symptoms which often closely resembled those of his nerve patients, and he was thus led to differentiate between the various symptoms, and to circumscribe them within their own limits. This was no easy matter; for he found not only that hysteria was liable to bring about every conceivable physical and mental disturbance, but also that its symptoms were often characterised by considerable variability. They would suddenly be called to life by events of many kinds, particularly of an emotional character, only to disappear with equal rapidity after a certain time. The symptoms of hysteria are manifold, and a few instances must suffice. They may be of a mild nature, such as headache, fatigue, lack of appetite, and spleen; or they may take a more serious turn and appear as grave physical disturbances, such as acute pain, complete or partial paralysis, persistent coughing fits and hiccoughs, blindness, deafness, dumbness and grave nerve attacks. The mental disturbances are primarily of an emotional character. The emotions are violent and impulsive, irrational and very variable. They may lead to a state of deranged excitability, and reach such a pitch that the patient appears to be insane. He may act as in a dream, and afterwards lose all recollection of his actions. All these symptoms were closely examined by Charcot and his pupils, but it was not found possible to localise the disturbances in any definite part of the spine or the brain. The cause of the disease was therefore to be looked for elsewhere, and Charcot assumed that in such cases there was a deterioration of the whole nervous system, brought about by hereditary degeneration. Another important discovery made by Charcot with regard to hysterical symptoms was destined to form the basis of later investigations. In cases of hysterical paralysis, he observed that he could arbitrarily bring about paralysis when the patient was in a hypnotic condition. At that time hypnosis was not a scientifically established fact, and such practices were despised as being primarily the methods of spiritualists and quacks. Charcot attempted to throw clearer light on the matter, although in the main he did not go much beyond describing numerous peculiarities of hypnosis and of the method by which it was induced; and he only made use of hypnosis for purposes of experiment, being unaware of its utility in treatment A big step forward was made later on by Liebault and Bernheim, who employed hypnosis to influence the symptoms of hysteria. They considered that since it was possible to bring about these symptoms during hypnotic sleep, it ought to be equally possible to remove them in that condition. Their hypothesis was verified. When hypnotised patients were spoken to in the proper manner, it was found that their symptoms could be influenced to a considerable degree. This discovery led to the further theory that, if any idea was impressed upon the mind of a hypnotised patient, it would be accepted without the slightest resistance. The process was called suggestion; and the mind of a hysterical patient was held to be more open to suggestion than that of a normal person. It further appeared that such suggestions were not only accepted, but that they exercised considerable influence on the entire physical and mental condition of the patient. To suggest that an arm was paralysed was enough to make it completely immovable; the suggestion of wine induced in the hypnotised person a condition apparently identical with drunkenness. It was inferred that both the symptoms of hysteria, and the paralysed or drunken condition were brought about in the self-same manner; the only difference being that, in the case of the disease, there was no hypnotist to induce the suggestion. It was therefore assumed that a similar suggestion could arise in the patient himself, caused either by a very powerful impression or by a deeply-stirring event. This was called auto-suggestion, and the receptive condition of the mind of such patients was defined as 'increased suggestibility'. It should be noted that this conception involves the curious implication that these suggestions are present in the patient's mind without his being aware of them in any way.

In France these questions were further examined very thoroughly and scientifically by Janet, one of Charcot's pupils. Various experiments, which led to a better insight into the psychology of hysteria, were made by him upon a number of patients, and it was found possible to establish beyond a doubt the existence of these unconscious processes of auto-suggestion. It was discovered that patients in deep hypnotic sleep were able to reply to questions, and so throw light on events in their earlier life, which were an important cause of their morbid symptoms. Thus unaccountable fits of dread occurring in a hysterical patient whenever she saw fire, were caused by a terrifying incident during a conflagration of which she had no conscious remembrance. Under hypnosis, she was able to relate the event with a wealth of detail. Another means of enquiring into the contents of the unconscious mind was afforded by automatic writing. When hysterical patients were given paper and pencil and their attention was distracted by random talk, the hand would often start writing and communicating facts that had no connection whatever with the subject of the conversation. If anyone approached the patient unnoticed from behind and whispered a question into his ear, it was not unusual for the patient to continue talking quite naturally, while his hand would write the reply. Thus even while the patient was not in a hypnotic trance, information could be elicited from him concerning details bearing upon his symptoms; and the fact was again clearly established that the unconscious retained these details, which were entirely inaccessible to the conscious memory. At times it was as if, behind the diseased personality of the patient, there was another being, much more fully cognisant of previous experiences. As a matter of fact, there have been well-known cases where a second personality has arisen into consciousness, such as that of the patient who had lost all recollection of a certain portion of her life, and whose symptoms obstructed several of her mental and physical faculties. By means of hypnosis another personality was evoked which could remember the forgotten period, and also possessed those faculties, but was unable to recollect anything else. It was even possible at times to conjure up another more complete personality, uniting in one whole the experiences and faculties of the two others. But such cases of double personality are very rare, and of little importance for our purpose, except in so far as they show that hysterical symptoms are caused by unconscious processes which have a more or less independent existence. They may best be compared with the so-called post-hypnotic suggestions, which are made to a hypnotised patient to be acted upon during waking hours. When such a suggestion is carried out at a given moment, the patient is at a loss to understand how he came to act in so strange a fashion.

But the problem of how such unconscious processes arise, is not yet solved. Is there something exceptional in the suggestion itself which compels it to remain unconscious, or does it depend entirely on the peculiar state of mind of the hysterical patient? And if so, what are the characteristics of this state? We may observe that normal people also are more or less susceptible to suggestions, but they are far from accepting all ideas as suggestions. In some psychological conditions, suggestibility can be greatly increased by more or less eliminating criticism in the patient. The personality of the suggestor is an important factor, and if recognised as an authority, he will have much more chance of enforcing his ideas without question. When the individual forms part of a crowd, he will also be more inclined to accept something on authority. Usually however in the minds of normal individuals different ideas are at work at the same time, checking and correcting each other. But suggestions made during hypnosis appear to develop quite independently in the mind ; they evolve and operate untrammelled by other ideas, and this occurs to a much greater extent with hysterical patients than with normal individuals. Hence Janet's characterisation of the hysterical state of mind as one in which ideas tend to subsist in watertight compartments. In his view, as in Charcot's, this is due to the general condition of the nervous system, which is the outcome of hereditary degeneration. In such cases it is much more difficult for one idea to affect another, because the mind of the degenerate has difficulty in retaining different ideas at the same time. Memory, according to Janet, arises from one idea evoking another, and if this connecting faculty is lacking, it is impossible for one idea to summon another into the conscious mind, and the apparent loss of memory of a particular event is thereby explained. Only under hypnosis can these dead memories be brought back to life by the hypnotist. Now an unconscious idea is just as well capable of influencing the body as conscious ideas do. Indeed an unconscious idea is even more operative, because it is not tempered by the workings of other ideas. Thus the unconscious recollection of a terrible conflagration may strike terror in the mind of the patient when he sees a tiny flame. Let us take as another example (XXI, p. 248) * the curious case of a patient who would sit down to table with a normal appetite, only to find that her hunger disappeared after the first mouthful and was immediately followed by repug-

* The Roman characters refer to the bibliography at the end of the book.

nance. She could give no reason for this, and only hypnosis revealed the still living recollection of a scene with her mother, who during a quarrel had upbraided her with not being worth the food she consumed, and said that she deserved to starve. This isolated unconscious idea rose up whenever she was about to eat, and affected her physical condition so violently as to dispel all appetite. By acting upon the unconscious idea during hypnosis, Janet succeeded in eliminating the symptom.

Janet's theory, no doubt, explains various characteristics of hysteria, but it leaves a number of questions unanswered. His patients were for the most part quite uneducated and mentally deficient women, so it was natural for him to attribute their psychological peculiarities to inferiority and degeneration. But hysterical symptoms very often occur in people who could certainly not be described as inferior, and do not make the impression of being able to retain only one idea at the same time. Janet also fails to make it clear why some ideas more than others tend to remain unconscious. It is true that he points to the influence exercised by strong emotions; but we shall see that all strong emotions are not to the same degree the cause of unconscious processes. One might also criticise Janet's association theory, according to which these processes consist of ideas which call each other forth because they are connected by association.

These objections were further elaborated by Breuer and Freud (VI), who at about the same time were pursuing the study of hysteria in Vienna. Breuer was a medical practitioner, who in the course of his practice met with a curious experience. He was treating a hysterical girl who had nursed her father through a serious illness, during which she developed ever increasing symptoms of mental disease, until in the end, after her father's death, she became almost constantly afflicted with a strange disorder. Her right arm was rigid and insensitive, and although she could still quite well understand German, her mother tongue, she was only able to speak English. Breuer observed accidentally that her condition improved for several hours when, in her dream-like state, she related her harassing ideas and illusions ; so by way of treatment he made her talk for some time every evening, while she was in this state. The illusions which obsessed her were mostly connected with her father's illness, and memories of that period came back to her with photographic distinctness, accompanied by the distress which they had aroused. He now made the quite unexpected discovery that a hysterical symptom would disappear as soon as she had recalled and described, in her somnambulistic condition, the first occasion when the symptom occurred. This was always accompanied by violent expressions of emotion ; and she usually had first to relate a series of incidents during which the symptoms had appeared, before she was able to tell of the event which had originally provoked it, which was as follows. One evening she was anxiously watching over her invalid father, while expecting the arrival of a consulting surgeon. She was sitting by the bed, her right arm over the back of her chair. She began to imagine things very vividly, as she was wont to, and saw a black snake that was crawling down the wall towards her father, as if with the intention of biting him. She wanted to ward off the animal, but her right arm which hung over the back of the chair was numb, insensitive and rigid, and when she looked at her fingers they changed into small snakes with death's-heads. Then the serpent hallucination left her, and in her terror she attempted to pray, but found no words, except an English nursery rhyme, and could only think and pray in English. After this incident these reactions of stiffness in the arm and speaking in English recurred whenever she was seized with fear, and finally they became permanent. As soon as the patient became conscious of what gave rise to them, the symptoms disappeared for good. Breuer found that this method succeeded in the case of her other morbid symptoms too. He communicated these facts to Freud, who made similar experiments on various patients. He found that the most varied forms of hysteria could be made to disappear by inducing the patient to relate the psychical moment which had given rise to them, provided that the emotions associated with these memories were also adequately expressed. It thus became apparent that patients in their normal consciousness knew nothing of these past events, that these recollections only emerged under hypnosis, and then very vividly. Breuer and Freud inferred that the psychic content can be at the same time both unconscious and operative, and they agreed with Janet in regarding the splitting up or dissociation of the mind as a marked characteristic of hysteria.

So far the investigations of both schools had attained the same results. But while Janet strove to alleviate hysterical symptoms by altering or eliminating under hypnosis the unconscious ideas which were at the basis of them, Breuer and Freud aimed at bringing out and expressing the emotional incidents which had caused these unconscious ideas, in order to render their action inoperative. They were thus led to examine closely the circumstances attending the origin of these unconscious morbid ideas. Their attention was soon directed towards a new phenomenon, which had already appeared in the Breuer case, and became increasingly noticeable during Freud's subsequent investigations: the repression at the critical moment of the powerful emotion which was always connected with these morbid ideas. Breuer's patient had not been able to express her concern and anxiety in the presence of her sick father, and so was compelled to conceal her real feelings. In another case, that of an employee, hysteria arose after he had been abused and struck in the street by his employer, a painful situation during which he had had to repress his feelings. Most of the examples given by Freud in his first work are too complicated to be quoted here. Very often morbid symptoms are not caused by one particular event, but by the repeated repression of the same emotion. Such repression indicates that in these cases there is a conflict between different emotions.

This theory of repression was confirmed by another experiment. In milder cases of hysteria, Freud found himself unable to hypnotise his patients for the purpose of discovering unconscious ideas. He then remembered that there was another method of penetrating to the unconscious memory. He had witnessed Bernheim's success in making a patient remember what had happened to her under hypnosis, although she had previously forgotten everything about it, simply by impressing upon her that it would come back to her when he put his hand upon her forehead. Freud's first experiment was to make the same gesture of the hand while he told his patient that he would remember something connected with the first appearance of his symptoms. When this had been repeated several times, memories were actually evoked, which gradually came nearer to the event which Freud was looking for. But at the same time, it became clear, not only to Freud but to the patient, that something was resisting this attempt to draw the recollection into the conscious mind, and that it was only by an effort that he could bring himself to speak of things which awakened unpleasant feelings. A *resistance* had to be overcome. This resistance also expressed a conflict of emotions. Freud concluded that the resistance which he had met with during treatment must have been the original cause for the disappearance of the past event from consciousness. Not only the condition of the patient, but also the reason for the repression, became more easy to understand. What had characteristically happened to this hysterical patient, was that a morbid symptom had taken the place of the emotional recollection which had been thrust back. Breuer and Freud explained this by saying that in place of one physical expression of emotion, another physical expression had arisen, a process which they called the *conversion* of an emotion into a morbid symptom. Such conversion of an unexpressed emotion could be terminated by bringing about its normal expression, or in technical language, by " allowing the affect to be worked off."

The following example will make the matter clearer.

I was treating a seventeen year old girl, who was suffering from a hiccough which had been tormenting her continuously for several weeks. She was quite at a loss to explain how it began, and no physical cause of the disturbance could be discovered. When I urged her to confide to me what was occupying her thoughts, she began describing her home conditions. After her father's death her mother had opened a boarding-house, which she was helping to run, and they had so far succeeded in keeping the household together for her brothers. When I continued to urge her, she related the small troubles of her life in the boarding-house and other matters concerning her brothers, and memories came back of an earlier time when her father was alive. After a few days, pauses began to occur in her story; she would refuse to go on, and became out of humour without being able to explain why. In proportion as it grew more difficult for her to express her thoughts, she became more restless and depressed, and would sometimes break out into fits of crying. She began to resist my questioning, and after a time the resistance became very marked. She told me with great difficulty about various disagreements with her mother, and thought she could remember that something of that kind had preceded the first fit of hiccoughs. Then at last, after further serious difficulties and more crying, the conscious recollection arose of the scene that had taken place just before she became afflicted with hiccoughs. Her mother had told her that the boarding-house was becoming too much for her: she proposed to give it up and to go and live with some relations. Her daughter was to look out for a situation. This was a heavy blow to the girl, who was very much attached to the family circle; and that evening after hearing of the plan, she gave way to bitter crying, and her sobs were so violent that they broke out convulsively like hiccoughs. At last she fell asleep. When she awoke the next morning, she had lost all recollection of the conversation, and, instead, was suffering from a continuous hiccough, which was so loud as to be very troublesome both to herself and to her family. Thus she had succeeded in thrusting away a painful memory; but although it had become unconscious, it now found indirect expression, as a kind of symbol for the hidden unhappiness. The treatment consisted in overcoming the resistance; and as soon as that was effected, the hiccough disappeared once and for all, and the girl's unhappiness expressed itself more normally in bitter tears. I should add for the sake of completeness, that in this case there was no reason for assuming the existence of any kind of hereditary degeneration. The patient was an intelligent, sensible girl, who had previously shown no symptoms of nervous disease; so that we may assume that in this case the troubles were serious enough to bring about the morbid symptoms.

After his first investigations with Breuer, Freud pursued his enquiries alone, and soon realised that his theoretic conceptions needed amplification. If hysterical symptoms usually occur whenever there has been repression, one would surely expect them to occur more frequently. Does not civilisation compel us every day to repress our emotions, and are they not frequently of a violent character? This, then, is not enough to explain how hysterical symptoms arise. Freud discovered that it was not always the repression of strong emotions that was the cause of morbid symptoms. Sometimes they would appear with relatively small occasion. But in such cases he found that there were always a great many previous experiences of the same nature, which together constituted a conflict in the patient's emotional life. For instance, (VI) he found that mild hysterical symptoms occurred in a governess in consequence of a scolding from the master of the house. Further investigation revealed a few other small matters, which all touched the patient on one sensitive spot, where her feelings were in conflict. She had been entrusted with the care of some children, whose mother was dead; and certain expressions of the father had given her the idea that she might some day become his second wife. But she repressed these thoughts, and found support for this repression in some of the father's less friendly utterances. This is a case where a lingering and chronic conflict may be considered the cause of mild morbid symptoms.

While investigating the problem why such conflicts should have such unusually far-reaching effects, Freud was led to penetrate more and more into the life history of his patients. It appeared that no single event that had at some time or other called forth a hysterical symptom, was sufficient in itself to explain this result. In his patients' antecedents there were always to be found various occurrences, which had provoked an inner conflict, and created the sensitive spot where the later event was to strike home. Thus, in the hiccough case referred to above, the painful problem had already arisen earlier in the young girl's life. Ever since the death of her father, she must have been always more or less conscious of the threatened break-up of the family household.

The antecedents of his patients became an increasingly important and fruitful field for Freud's investigations. But he found that at a certain moment in the treatment of a patient, his recollections would cease, and that then he had already reached back to the events of early childhood. Even at this early stage of emotional life, he would at times find peculiarities which had developed later on into conflicts of emotion. It seemed as though certain future characteristics could be ascribed entirely to some earlier experience which had powerfully impressed itself upon the mind. It sometimes also appeared that a conflict of emotions had existed very early in life, and had led to concealment and repression. At first Freud considered these events of early childhood, which had led to conflict and repression, to be actually the predisposing causes of mental disease, especially of hysteria. But he soon abandoned this view, when further investigation showed that many normal people had had similar conflicts in early youth, which yet had not resulted in morbid conditions in later life. Furthermore he discovered that in a few cases the deeply stirring event in childhood had not in fact taken place at all, but only existed in the child's vivid imagination. The main cause of a morbid disposition should not be exclusively sought for in the event which had acted as an outer stimulus to certain emotions in the child. We must suppose either that there was something peculiar in the child which made it more susceptible to the unfavourable influence of certain events, or that the child had experienced a conflict of emotions solely through its imagination. These deviations, which lead to hysterical symptoms, are not therefore provoked by circumstance alone, but also by disposition. The value of Freud's enquiry was certainly not impaired by this revised conception, for he was able to show how disposition is developed and influenced by all manner of circumstances, and how morbid symptoms receive their specific form and content through the interaction of disposition and outward events.

Meanwhile Freud was drifting further and further away from his earlier adherence to association-psychology. We have seen how near he originally was to Janet, who considered that certain unconscious images were the active forces which caused such morbid symptoms. According to this psychological theory, ideas constitute the essential part of the mind. They attract and repel each other like atoms in the physical world, and our judgments and convictions are the outcome of their interactions. Breuer and Freud saw at once that these active forces of the mind lay not so much in the ideas, as in the emotions that were connected with them and gave them their importance. If we follow Freud's method and look back into the past history of a human being, we become more and more aware that life is flowing on continuously like a stream, in which the emotions seem to be always changing, though in essence they remain the same, however much they may clothe themselves in new ideas. By thus viewing a man's life as a whole, we can penetrate deeper and deeper into regions that lie behind ideas. The emotions give clear evidence of this deeper background, for they reveal definite currents which, however mingled and shifting, are yet an indication of certain fixed desires. We must finally regard these underlying desires, which express themselves in emotions and thoughts, as the ultimate basis of our mental life. In youth, these impulses express themselves more simply and vaguely, but later on in a more involved fashion. They then split up, or unite together, and tend to become more differentiated, and at the same time more complicated and more pronounced. But however far back into our lives we project our memory, we never find any singleness of aim in our desires. Already in our earliest years we discover conflicts of emotion, expressing forces which clash with one another. These conflicts become conscious as emotional reactions of many different kinds.

While investigating cases of mental disturbances, Freud observed the curious fact that the ideas and emotions which were repressed in hysterical cases, all belonged to the same extensive category, that of sex. In the expression of sexual emotions, there was always some disturbance to be noted. Hysterical symptoms had taken the place of the normal forms of expression. We may at first be tempted to connect this view with the popular conception that hysteria and sexual excitement are one and the same thing. It is an old theory, as is shown by the name, which is derived from the Greek word for womb. Hysteria was principally to be found in women, and its symptoms were therefore connected with sexual deviations. Freud's theory confirms this view only in so far as it makes clear that hysterical symptoms are a substitute for and a disguised expression of sexual impulses, which for one reason or another have not been able to express themselves as such. Now and then hysterical patients show strong sexual desires quite clearly. But just because the normal expressions of sexual desire have been involuntarily repressed, there can generally be no question at all of sexual excitement in the ordinary sense. On the contrary, such patients are cold and detached, although there may sometimes be indications showing that they are capable of sexual emotion. However that may be, I hope to have shown clearly that hysteria and sexual excitement are not the same thing.

On the basis of Freud's authority and experience, we shall assume that hysterical symptoms often arise in a complicated manner, which the patient himself cannot account for, as the result of repressed sexual emotions, the term sexual being used in a very general sense. Without entering into detail, it may be well to delineate the various factors which produce hysteria. For the sake of convenience, we shall distinguish between three kinds of hysteria, and consider the origin of each in turn.

We have seen that both past and present circumstances are of importance in bringing about morbid symptoms. In cases of obvious predisposition, the emphasis should be placed on previous incidents and circumstances as having prepared the later morbid reactions. In genuine hysterical cases significant characteristics exist even in early childhood, and, as Freud has shown, are caused by strong, unconscious emotions reacting upon the conscious life. At a very early period, whether owing to circumstance or disposition, strong erotic emotions find a form of expression, which is subsequently repressed. But this repression soon more or less miscarries, so that the influence of the unconscious makes itself felt, though in a concealed manner. This influence especially shows itself in over-tension of the emotions, leading to violent outbursts about trifles, unaccountable terrors and other morbid feelings, and often taking the form of a demonstrativeness unusual at that age. Such children are likely to be unusually sympathetic, sensitive and unselfish, but at the same time they show themselves to be as changeable in their sentiments as adult patients. In later life unexpected influences constantly intervene and disturb their relations with others, so that they gain the reputation of being exacting, difficult, jealous and intolerant. They are also blamed for attitudinising, for they are so anxious to make an impression on their entourage, that they do not scruple to mix fact and fiction. It will often be remarked how different the rôle they wish to impersonate, is from the one which they usually express in their actions. This is due to the emergence of their unconscious processes, which are much more noticeable to onlookers than to the patients themselves, who owing to their repressions are not able to become conscious of them. In fact their attention is only drawn to these processes, when they assume the form of troublesome hysterical symptoms. Even then their connection with the other workings of the mind is generally so little apparent, that patients will only become convinced of it after special efforts of introspection. Just as small difficulties and conflicts produced unaccountable and disproportionate emotional reactions, so these reactions lead to more or less pronounced morbid symptoms, which may seem equally mysterious in their origin. In serious cases, these symptoms may dominate the whole of the patient's life; and as they are generally accompanied by peculiar emotional reactions, he is likely to become very difficult to deal with.

A careful observer will note a peculiar attitude in such patients towards the general question of sex and love. Everything in this sphere that is not exclusively and definitely spiritual, is rejected as inferior. The patient will behave as if he were far above such problems and conflicts; but various details of behaviour, his curiosity, and certain unmistakeable reactions will show that he is very far indeed from being uninterested in such questions, and that unconsciously he is more interested in them than most other people. As a result he will often be misunderstood, for it will not be realised how little his involuntary behaviour corresponds to his conscious intention.

So far we have dealt with patients, whose mental deviations have extended over so long a time, that the causes must be looked for in congenital disposition or in events of early childhood. We now come to a second category, that of patients who become afflicted with hysteria at a certain moment in their lives, as a result of some critical difficulty. In cases of this kind it is easier to discover the causes of the disease, as they are much more in evidence. It is true that here also an enquiry into character and disposition would reveal emotions, which at an earlier period have been thrust back into the unconscious. But the repression will have been less comprehensive, and more successful, and more outlets will have been found for impulses and feelings, so that the severe tension caused by bottled-up emotions will never have expressed itself in a troublesome manner. In such a case the causes of morbid symptoms are in general unsatisfied desires in the emotional life. The symptoms appear when the emotions are debarred from a satisfactory outlet It might be objected that the patient might find other forms of expression; also that there are plenty of unsatisfied people who show no hysterical symptoms.

But to produce these symptoms, other conditions, connected with the tendency to repression, must be present. An unsatisfied desire causes strong mental tension and compression of emotional energy, and a number of older, elementary forms of expression crop up involuntarily. As the water of a dammed-up river is pressed back and flows into long abandoned channels, so the emotional tension will try to express itself in obsolete forms. Old habits, events or fantasies, which were accompanied in the past by strong emotion, will emerge once more as possible outlets for the suppressed emotion. This process is called *regression,* and occurs also in normal people; but with them it is more consciously developed than with hysterical patients, who not only would never consciously adopt earlier ways of expression, but cannot even conceive them as a possible outlet.

In many cases normal persons are able to find new forms of expression, when the old have to be given up. A girl who is unfortunate in love may find satisfaction in nursing; a writer can express his unsatisfied ideal of love in a novel. Everyone does not possess to an equal degree this capacity for transferring sex feeling into channels of greater social value, a process which Freud calls *sublimation.* In most people it soon reaches its limits. In hysterically disposed individuals, the tendency to repress and the refusal to face facts about themselves, make it more difficult both to discover the trouble and to find a possible solution through sublimation, and so the unconscious tension is increased.

Whereas in the first group of hysterical cases the tendency to repress rouses strong unconscious activities continuously throughout the patient's life, in the second series the unconscious only emerges in a troublesome manner when a want has to go unsatisfied, so that a tension arises and seeks an outlet which is denied. This tension in its turn produces a regression towards earlier forms of expression; but they are unable to penetrate into consciousness, and so the tension has to find an abnormal outlet.

In a third series of cases, a hysterical symptom will suddenly appear in connection with an unusually severe shock, or with some emotion, which has either not been expressed at all, or only inadequately. In the war, such cases were very common. Here too investigation will generally reveal a predisposition to hysteria; but it will not be an overwhelming factor, as in the two previous groups. Such cases are easier to cure than the others, for it is easier to bring back to consciousness the disturbing event, and to provoke the proper expression of the emotion.* Where the tendency to repression has become a settled habit, and frustrates partly or completely the expression of important impulses, the treatment presents much greater difficulty. The patient can no doubt find some relief by pouring out his innermost feelings to somebody in whom he places his trust. But if this method were

* Unless the symptom acquires a secondary use which induces the patient to cling to it later on, *e.g.* fear of the trenches.

the only one used, it would lead the patient to be too dependent on his doctor. The repressed emotions will, it is true, find a different outlet from that provided by morbid symptoms ; but when the treatment comes to an end, and this mode of expression is no longer possible, the patient will probably relapse sooner or later, and again become subject to the same or other morbid symptoms.

Thus a double problem confronts the psycho-analyst, when he has to deal with the more serious forms of hysteria. In the first place he must discover the seat of the various repressed emotions, and their connection with the morbid symptoms. Next, the patient must be induced to give up the bad habit of repressing his difficulties, and be taught how to find better outlets for his emotions by introspection, and by giving thought to his troubles, and so will learn how to direct his life in a more conscious manner. Small wonder that when the symptoms date from far back, or where individual characteristics are strongly pronounced, the treatment becomes a lengthy and difficult affair. It is only when the patient has abandoned the comfortable position of refusing to see things as they are, and has come to face realities within and without, that he is able to find satisfaction for his emotional needs. Until then, his utterances of repressed emotions in the presence of the doctor are only a safety valve for the tension of his emotional energy ; and so long as this lasts, the patient remains more or less dependent on his doctor. But the doctor should always make his patients realise the nature of their dependence on him ; and this he can do by making them see that their unconscious infantile emotions are thus being satisfied. It is obvious that such a treatment must make severe demands on the analyst. He will have to retain an objective attitude towards the most variegated emotions of his patient, neither rejecting them, nor accepting them, and he must reflect all his utterances faithfully like a mirror. Psycho-analytical treatment essentially consists in the attainment by the patient of fundamental self-knowledge by systematic and lengthy introspection. Opportunities for investigating inner problems will be furnished not only by the more or less important morbid symptoms, but by innumerable forms of expression which have no apparent connection with our conscious mental life. In a later chapter, I hope to show how some of these phenomena occur in normal persons too, and may give us insight into the unconscious. In psycho-analytical treatment dreams provide very important clues for penetrating into the depths of the unconscious.

I do not intend here to make a profound study of the problems of psycho-pathology. Besides, it would be difficult to summarise briefly the various processes by which hysterical symptoms are connected with earlier incidents and fancies in the patient's life. But it may be as well to state now emphatically, what I hope to prove later on, that our mental life is far more complicated, composite and mysterious than most of us suppose on the strength of a superficial knowledge of our own conscious processes. We are ever ready with opinions about ourselves and others, and with the offer of advice to all and sundry. A better understanding of the complex structure of the human mind will make us tread more warily. Psycho-analysts, who are daily confronted with these problems, are all well aware of their overwhelming difficulty, which puts a strain upon all their faculties. Anyone who undertakes the psycho-analytical treatment of a patient without adequate preparation, has no right to ascribe failure simply to the method of treatment. It should also be clear that this treatment, more than any other, requires the co-operation of the patient. Understanding can only be attained if patient and doctor constantly work hand in hand; and unless patients are really anxious to be cured, and are prepared to investigate themselves thoroughly, they are unsuitable for this kind of treatment.

We must now consider this further question. A patient may repress his impulses because they are unacceptable to him, or because they clash with the rest of his emotions. He will have to find some serviceable forms of expression for his emotions by becoming more conscious of his inner life. But is this always possible? May it not happen that either his emotional disposition, or his incapacity to create useful sublimated forms of expression, are of such a kind that the attempt to make him realise his problems may merely torture him without solving his difficulties? Would it not be better to leave his morbid symptoms undisturbed, rather than increase the difficulty of the conflict by making him acutely conscious of it? May not repression be a fortunate piece of mechanism?

We ought to differentiate between the various individual cases, and consider in each separately whether the advantages of treatment will outweigh the drawbacks. Generally the patient will be able to tell by intuition whether a psycho-analytical treatment will suit his inner powers and disposition. No serious psycho-analyst will force his treatment upon a patient. The liberty to break off the treatment at any time, and to carry on introspection by oneself, is of the first importance. But although there may at times be objections to treatment, they should not be overrated. Even in cases of an unfavourable disposition, a clear understanding of the difficulties, and a conscious effort to overcome them, will afford a much better chance of a solution than would a mere struggle in the dark.

I will now briefly summarise the results of our enquiry into hysteria. Charcot disposed of the conception that hysterical patients are female humbugs, who want to create an effect. It was left to his pupils to establish clearly that hysteria is connected with unconscious mental processes. So long as such processes were ascribed to an inferior mental disposition, the stigma of degeneracy was attached to anyone who showed hysterical symptoms. A change of view was brought about by Freud, who pointed out the importance of various influences which modify our emotional life from childhood onwards. Although hereditary disposition remains in many cases a factor of importance, in a great many others the emphasis should be placed on circumstances which have warped the growth of the emotions. Unconscious ideas and emotions are no longer considered to be by themselves the causes of the disease, but are looked upon as symptoms of repressed impulses, which would have found a satisfying outlet if other emotions had not intervened. The origin of hysteria may therefore be described as a conflict of vitally important impulses, which results in the repression of one among them.

Experience also proves that these repressed impulses are always connected with sex, this term being used in its widest sense. Thus the old connection between hysteria and sex has been re-established, but not in the sense that hysterical patients must be persons with strong sexual requirements. On the contrary, Freud has shown that such requirements are here repressed. The popular conception is only so far true, that sex is seen to crop up everywhere in the utterances of hysterical patients, because these repressed needs, of which the patient remains entirely unconscious, are always endeavouring indirectly to push themselves forward. It would be foolish to attempt the cure of such patients merely by providing them with direct sexual satisfaction. Not only would other emotions oppose this very strenuously, but the whole temper of their emotional life is too delicate and complex to find satisfaction in a coarse and elementary manner. What is needed is that by increasing the sphere of their consciousness, they should attain a new harmony of the emotions, which would not simply consist in rejecting what does not fit in with the whole. The path that leads to this harmony has been revealed by Freud's difficult and slow psycho-analytical treatment, which compels the patient to become conscious of himself by a careful investigation of the workings of his mind. The essence of this method is a long and systematic introspection, by which we may penetrate not only into what is generally called the unconscious, but also into those thoughts and emotions which can only be made conscious after some inner resistance has been laboriously overcome. It is only these last processes which Freud describes as unconscious, while he defines as pre-conscious processes such matters as can easily and without any resistance emerge into consciousness.

Freud's views on hysteria have now been accepted by many investigators, although there are still a number of doctors who adhere to the vague conception of hereditary degeneration without further inquiring into its causes. Meanwhile the new theories are percolating through, and have given us an entirely novel view of the nature of insanity, while the inner conflict between conscious personality and repressed unconscious tendencies plays an important part in general psycho-pathology. But this is a subject which is too complex for me to dwell upon in this book. Thus the study of hysteria and Freud's discovery of the psycho-analytical method have enabled us to penetrate by entirely new paths into the dark recesses of the human mind; and we have come to realise that it is a very complicated organism, of which only a small portion is known to us in the conscious processes of our daily life.

CHAPTER II

THE UNCONSCIOUS IN THE NORMAL MIND

We have seen that the study of neuroses, especially of hysteria, has led to an increased understanding of the unconscious processes. Freud has shown that there are two kinds of unconscious processes: the *pre-conscious*, of which one is not aware at any given moment, but which it is possible, more or less readily, to recall to consciousness; and the *repressed unconscious*, which consciousness resists, because it contains impulses which would not fit in with the rest of the personality.

We now come to the question: does the repressed unconscious play any part in normal people, or must we look for it only in the abnormal? We cannot give a complete answer if we rely merely on what we know about ourselves, because the very fact that there are unconscious processes in our mind, implies that we are not aware of them. But just as in hysterical cases we were led to admit the existence of unconscious feelings and thoughts, because of various symptoms which could not be explained by the conscious personality alone, so we can assume that there are unconscious processes in normal people, because in them also expressions occur which have no apparent relation to the conscious mind. Freud was naturally led to study these expressions, when investigating the psychic products of his patients. He found that not only morbid products could be traced back to unconscious origins, but also slight disturbances such as we frequently meet with in normal people, which are not usually classed among morbid symptoms. Instances of these are: forgetting names and foreign words, slips of the tongue or of the pen, forgetting what one meant to do, making slight mistakes and breaking objects, etc. Furthermore he found that dreams in particular showed the way to a clearer understanding of the unconscious, as they are the spontaneous experience of a mental state, in which conscious criticism and reflection are almost completely absent. A close study of all these symptoms, which occur also in normal people, will teach us a great deal about the content and significance of the normal unconscious processes.

We must first consider some of the disturbances of the conscious mind. Formerly these were explained by the fact that they are much more apt to occur when the mind is fatigued and distracted than when it is fresh and wide-awake. Although this is certainly true, it does not explain why a special disturbance arises at any given moment. Here Freud's theories give us a clue. He made his patients concentrate their attention each on some particular disturbance, and asked them to tell him all the thoughts that occurred to them. Freud attaches importance to all the thoughts that are thus naturally associated with a given phenomenon, even if the patient himself does not see any meaning in them. He found that when the search-light of the patient's attention had been fixed for some time on the moment of the disturbance, and various associated ideas had been called forth out of the dark background, it usually became clear that the disturbance was related to a conflict between the conscious thought and an unconscious feeling, which was not in harmony with it. In some cases this contrast was superficial and easily recognised, in other cases a strong resistance had to be overcome on the part of the patient in order to make him recognise it.

A few instances may serve as illustrations. A young man is engaged to a young lady of a somewhat angular character, with whom he is very much in love. He often calls her his angel, and thus describes her in a letter to a friend : " My fiancée is a perfect angle."

A patient made an unjustified attack upon me during treatment, and refused to see that she was in the wrong. When speaking of another doctor, she said, " I treated him also very badly." This " also " led her to recognise that she was in the wrong.

Another patient, to whom the payment of my fee was probably somewhat of an effort, said to me on leaving : " I have no money with me to-day to pay your fee, but I will forget it next time."

Prof. Bleuler relates the following instance of misreading (IV, p. 121). " Once, while reading, I had the curious feeling that I had seen my name printed two lines further down. To my astonishment I only found the word 'Blutkörperchen' (blood-corpuscles). This is the strongest instance of misreading I have ever met with among the many thousand cases which I have analysed. If ever I thought I saw my name, the real word usually resembled it much more strongly, and in most cases it contained at least all the letters of my name. However, in this case the relation to myself which caused the optical illusion was quite clear. I was reading at that moment the conclusion of a passage containing a criticism of a certain kind of bad style in scientific work, of which I felt guilty myself."

Dr Stekel relates the following instance of a slip of the pen (VIII, p. 66). "Somebody had accused the editor of a well-known weekly paper of being corruptible, and an article had to be written in defence of the editor. This was done with great enthusiasm. The chief editor of the paper read the article; the author of course read it both in manuscript and in proof, and they all passed it. Finally the proof-reader's turn comes, and he points out a small mistake which they have all missed. The sentence ran: 'our readers must admit that we have always represented the general interest in the most selfish way.' Of course the word 'unselfish' was intended, but the real thought broke through the eloquent appeal with irresistible force."

A matron in a hospital had to fill in upon some form the name of a patient who had just died. She suddenly noticed that she was writing the name of another patient from an adjoining ward. The names began with the same letter. But this other patient, who was still alive, was a specially difficult one, and was always wanting to do forbidden things; so it was no wonder that the matron wished to get rid of him.

The following instance came to me from a very reliable source. A doctor in hospital had a great dislike to a certain nurse, because she often severely criticised some of his actions. On one occasion this nurse was unwell and he had to prescribe for her. He wrote out the prescription for a tonic called ferratine, and he was very surprised when the chemist sent the prescription back with the message that he must have made a mistake. He had written instead of ferratine " veratrine " which is such a deadly poison that it hardly ever occurs in prescriptions. In this case the doctor would find it hard to admit that his dislike of the nurse was expressed in such a forcible manner. But we must remember that the unconscious expresses itself in a much more narrow and violent form when its expression is unmodified by the conscious feelings.

Many of us have had the experience of taking a latchkey out of our pocket when we are passing a friend's house, and have usually found that it was a house where we felt thoroughly at home. Again when we leave an umbrella or walking-stick at somebody's house, we may assume that it means that we would like to return there. In order to be absolutely certain of such an explanation, it would of course be necessary for us to examine whether there really was such a motive at the bottom of our feelings. Psycho-analysis has drawn attention to many of these occurrences, and an increasing number of instances are now known.

The psycho-analyst Dr Sachs relates how he twice made the same mistake of going up too many flights of stairs in a building of flats. The first time he found that he was lost in a day-dream about climbing into a higher social status. The second time he realised that he was worrying at the time about some criticism of his work, in which he had been attacked for going " too far." His unconscious thoughts had thus been automatically translated into a symbolic action.

An interesting mistake was made by a lady who

suffered from a weak digestion, and had to follow a severe diet. Her husband was carving a delicious piece of roast meat which she was forbidden to eat, and asked her to pass the mustard. The lady went to the sideboard, and got out something which she put before her husband, without noticing that it was her medicine (VIII).

Probably many people will have noticed that they are apt to lose or break a present when they have quarrelled with the donor. When once we have turned our attention to these matters, it is often easy to find such reasons for little disturbances. But sometimes it is more difficult ; and such trifles may occasionally be the disguise of serious inner conflicts. It may even occur that an unexpected awkwardness resulting in an accident, must be ascribed to unconscious suicidal thoughts.

We should be on our guard against attaching an unconscious significance to all disturbances of this kind in other people, because they may arise from such a variety of sources, and we may very easily be mistaken. The most fruitful method is to study such symptoms in ourselves, as our material there lies close to hand. It is only when we know people extremely well that we can guess what is the background of these slight mistakes.

The significance of dreams is usually much more difficult to understand than that of such small disturbances ; though sometimes we meet with very transparent dreams, of which the following is an instance. A coquettish good-looking young girl told how she was sitting in her dream by the edge of some water in which great fishes were swimming. Her beautiful fair hair was in one long plait, finished off with a scarlet bow ; she was dangling this in the water, and fishes kept coming up to bite the plait, and then disappeared again. At last one was caught and landed, when to her surprise it turned into a young man of her acquaintance.

This kind of dream, which probably everyone will explain in the same way, is very rare in comparison with the enigmatical ones ; and hence the conviction had grown up that dreams are merely deceiving, fantastical images which arise by chance during sleep. In former times they were looked upon from a very different point of view, and the instances of dream interpretation in the Bible are good illustrations of the significance ascribed to them by all ancient peoples. A prince would consult his dreams before undertaking a hazardous expedition. Dreams were believed to reveal the cause and cure of illnesses. They were held to be the inspirations of gods or demons ; and a special meaning was ascribed to certain signs in the dream, which could only be interpreted by priests or "medicine-men," and were collected later on in dream books. Nowadays all this is regarded as mere superstition, and most people will feel reluctant to begin again ascribing meanings to dreams.

Freud's theory of dreams, however, is very far removed from these ancient ideas. He does not search the dream for prophecies or information from outside the dreamer's own mind, but uses it only as a means of penetrating into his inner life, by discovering the relation of the dream to his experiences and recollections. He does not therefore explain every image in the dream arbitrarily, but makes the patient think of any ideas that may occur to him in connection with some particular image, and which might explain why it arose. If for instance a house occurs in a dream, Freud does not ask, " What do you think is the meaning of this house ? " but he requests the patient to fix his whole attention on the image of the house, and to consider whether he has ever seen it before, or whether perhaps it reminds him of some other house. In this way the dreamer will not have to concern himself with the possible inter-relation of the various images in the dream ; and it will be found that this is the way we all naturally set about to look for the origin of a mental image. We ask ourselves : " how did I get that image ? Where did I hear or see such a thing before ? " When we have thus found various ideas, that are related to the images in the dream, we shall then have a network of associated ideas which are usually related to each other at various points of junction. This inter-relation is of great importance, and will help to throw light on many obscurities in the dream.

In order to understand the meaning of dreams, it is best to begin with simple ones, such as those of children, which do not require any deep analysis. Freud gives some good instances of these (XV, p. 133). A little boy of two years old was made to offer a basket of cherries to someone. He probably felt this as a great sacrifice, and the next morning he told his dream in the following words : " Hermann eaten up all the cherries." A little girl of three years old was allowed to go in a boat on the lake for the first time. She enjoyed herself so much that she would not leave the boat, and cried when she was taken out. The next morning she said : " Last night I was going on the lake in a boat."

These children's dreams show clearly how desires, which have not been satisfied, or only partially, the day before, may be realised in dream. This also applies to the dreams of people who are suffering from physical needs, such as explorers suffering from thirst, who dream of great stretches of water. Nordenskjöld relates that the men who shared his winter quarters in the polar regions, were always dreaming of food and drink (XV, p. 140). Their dreams satisfied other desires as well, for one of them dreamt that the postman brought a large mail for them. In the same way a prisoner will dream about escape or freedom.

In the next class of dreams come those in which physical sensations or noises have been woven into the dream. We often notice that a fairly long dream has only lasted a very short time. The following dream for instance was the reaction to the sound of an alarum clock : (XV, p. 92). The dreamer goes out on a fine spring morning, and walks through the fields to a neighbouring village. He sees the villagers going to church in their Sunday clothes, and decides to join them ; but first he walks round the churchyard. While he is reading the inscriptions on the tombstones, he hears the bell-ringer ascending the tower, and he looks up at the church-bell which is going to be set in movement. At last he sees that it begins to move, and the sounds are so clear and strong that they wake him, and he finds that it is the sound of the alarum. It is probable that the mechanical sound, which precedes the actual ringing of the alarum, warned the sleeper, and so caused this dream, in which we see this expectant attitude reflected.

A Norwegian, Mourly Vold, has made a long series of experiments about this kind of dream, which is caused by an outside stimulus. One of his experiments was to pinch the dreamer's neck softly, who would then dream about a mustard plaster which had been applied to him as a child, and about the doctor who treated him at the time. If a drop of water was let fall on his forehead, he would dream that he was in Italy, perspiring from the heat.

Freud arrived at the conclusion, based on similar dreams, that dreams occur when an outer or an inner sense-stimulus threatens to disturb sleep. If the stimulus is woven into the dream, then sleep is not disturbed ; but the sleeper will be wakened if the stimulus is too strong. Freud therefore regards the dream as the guardian of sleep. He gives the remarkable instance of a medical student, who is called in the morning, because he must go to his work at the hospital, but falls asleep again, and dreams that he is lying in bed in one of the hospital's wards, and reflects that now he need not get up as he is already in the hospital (IX, p. 91).

Not all dreams however contain pleasant images ; on the contrary they may be full of fear or of other disagreeable ideas, and so cannot all be regarded, like children's dreams, as the realisation of some wish. The study of hysteria will throw some light on the interpretation of these unpleasant or indifferent dreams, since it has taught us that the human mind is full of conflicting emotions and desires. Even an apparently harmonious consciousness may have a background of discordant unconscious processes. Freud found that these unconscious thoughts and emotions were expressed much more clearly in dreams than in conscious life; but that even in dreams a certain restraining influence was hardly ever absent, by which these emotions were changed or disguised so that they could not be immediately recognised. Freud compared this process with the work of a censor, whose business it is to suppress the expression of certain thoughts and feelings. But one of the various ways of escaping a censorship, is to express one's thoughts in an indirect, disguised manner; and this is what happens in dreams. When Freud analysed his patients' dreams, and tried to overcome their resistance, the relation between these indirect expressions and certain unconscious desires was constantly brought to light. In connection with his theory that the dream is the guardian of sleep, he regarded these disguised dreams as a compromise between the repressed desires, which are trying to force a way out, and the repressing censor Therefore if sleep is disturbed in these cases, it is because the dreamer's wishes are not realised. It is not surprising that in cases of sharp mental conflict the rising up into consciousness of these repressed desires may cause much disturbance and anxiety to the dreamer.

Dreams of this kind occur in normal as well as abnormal people, and frequently contain even less disguise. We all know the dreams that seem to us as unpleasant because we cannot approve of their content; and we are all apt to dream things which we would rather not relate in public, even though no psycho-analyst were present.

But there is really no need to be afraid that a psycho-analyst might immediately deduce the most intimate secrets from a dream which he hears related; for he knows only too well by experience that dream-interpretation is a far too complicated affair, and that he could say little about a dream's significance without hearing the dreamer's associated thoughts. The danger lies more with outsiders, who have browsed a little in psycho-analytical books, and think they can interpret all dreams which they come across.

It is difficult to give a short yet complete instance of dream-analysis, because a dream is a complicated product related to all kinds of things in the dreamer's past and present life. The doctor will not only use the associated material for his analysis, but everything he knows about the patient's character and circumstances will help him to arrange this associated material into a comprehensive whole. Hence any instances I can give could never be so convincing as they are to the analyst or to the patient himself, who can always refer to the complete psychic background. It should also be remembered that it is very rare for one dream to be analysed by itself. Psycho-analytical treatment usually takes many months, during which time many dreams and other psychic expressions are examined. Naturally this has some influence on the character of the patient's dreams and thoughts. Things which are talked over during treatment may be redigested in a dream. I do not believe that the intrinsic nature of the dreams would be altered by thus directing the patient's attention to them; but in any case the whole process becomes much more complicated. In order to give a complete account of this, we should have to publish a whole series of dreams with all their associated material, and this would soon extend to the length of a long novel, and would contain many intimate details of the patient's life, which would not be permissible.

Notwithstanding these objections, I will try to give a few instances of dream-analysis. The first is the dream of a girl who had been under treatment for so short a time, that her mind had not yet been prejudiced by dream-theories. She dreamt that she read in the paper that a certain young man of her acquaintance had failed in his examination. She told me that the day before she had in fact looked in the paper to find the result of this examination, but had been unable to find it. If this young man passed, he would soon get married to a girl she rather disliked. She had the impression that his fiancée did not care for him enough, and did not behave well to him. After a good deal of further talk the fact emerged that she herself was much inclined to flirt with young men. All this helped to make the dream much clearer. It is probable that the failure in the examination was a disguise for the wish that the marriage should be prevented, because she was jealous of the fiancée.

Freud relates the following dream (XV, p. 127). A young woman, who had been married for several years, dreams that she is sitting in a theatre with her husband. One side of the stalls is quite empty. Her husband tells her that a friend of hers with her fiancée had also intended to come, but they had only been able to get very inferior seats, three for 1.50 kronen, and they thought this was not good enough. She thinks that it would not have been so bad. The apparent cause of the dream was the fact that her husband had told her that this friend of hers had become engaged. Also the week before she had been to a theatrical performance for which she had taken tickets very early, so that she had had to pay more for them. When she came to the theatre she had noticed how unnecessary her precaution had been, for one side of the stalls had been quite empty. Her husband had laughed at her for her unnecessary hurry. But what was the origin of the 1.50 kronen? She remembered that the day before she had heard that her sister-in-law had received 1.50 kronen from her husband, and that she had immediately spent it at a jeweller's. But why were there three tickets in the dream? The only thing that occurred to her in that connection is that her friend, who is just engaged, is only three months younger than herself, and she adds, "And yet I have already been married for ten years." Nothing further occurred to her in connection with the dream, but Freud could already interpret it with a fair amount of certainty. He was struck by the recurring motive of "too early" in the associated thoughts. She bought her tickets too early, and she condemned her sister-in-law for spending her money so soon. When he connected this with her saying that her friend had found a good husband, though she was only three months younger than herself, Freud suspected that the hidden feeling behind this dream was: "It was foolish of me to get married so early. My friend's case shows me that if I had waited, I could have found just as good a husband." Here therefore the marrying is disguised as going to a theatre. Space forbids me to say more about the symbolism of this dream, which would lead us into too many details.

A patient of Freud told a dream in which she had seen her sister's only son lying dead in his coffin, just as she had actually seen his elder brother, who had died a little time before (IX, p. 111). She maintained that this disproved Freud's theory that the dream expresses an unrealised wish, for she said that it was impossible for her to desire such a disaster. However after some enquiry the meaning of the dream was proved to be entirely different. She had formerly lived with this elder sister, and had made at that time the acquaintance of a professor, with whom she fell in love. Her sister however had prevented any engagement, and the professor had avoided meeting them since. But she was still in love with him and always attended his lectures, and she had meant to do so upon the day after the dream. When Freud asked her whether she could remember anything that happened after the death of her nephew, she said at once: "Yes, certainly. The professor came to call after a long interval, and we met again at the little coffin of my nephew." Inwardly she was resisting the desire to meet the object of her love, and therefore it was expressed in this very complicated way. If her nephew were to die, she might have another opportunity of meeting him.

Thus the interpretation of a dream aims at finding the *latent* content behind the apparent or *manifest* content. This *latent* content is the group of thoughts and emotions by which the dream is related to the mental life of the dreamer, and is therefore an integral part of the dreamer's mind. We discover the latent content by inducing the dreamer to let his mind dwell on the images of his dream, and record any impressions or thoughts that occur to him, without allowing any resistance or self-criticism to interfere. Freud has lately enlarged this technique considerably, because he has discovered the curious fact that there were certain dream-images, to explain which he was unable to collect any associated ideas, however much the dreamer might strive to overcome any possible resistance. Freud was led to translate these images in a new way, which was suggested to him by the symbolic meaning ascribed to them in popular language, proverbs and songs, and also in the symbolism of old myths and legends. His method has thus some resemblance to that which we find in the old dream-books. I must point out that Freud realised from the beginning that this form of interpretation might lead to dangerous misunderstandings, and repeatedly warned his pupils not to use this method except in certain special cases, and then only with the utmost caution. Freud wishes symbolic interpretation to be applied only to simple images of general human interest, such as the human body as a whole, parents, children, brothers and sisters, birth, death, nakedness and sexuality (XV, p. 164). The human body as a whole is often represented by a house, parents by royalties or persons in authority. Brothers and sisters are often symbolised as small animals or vermin: falling into water or being rescued from it, represents birth; dying is symbolised by setting out on a journey, or disappearing, nakedness by its opposite, clothes or uniform. According to Freud, sexual symbolism is very rich in its variety, and he gives a great many instances in his book.

At first these dream symbols will give the impression of being chosen quite arbitrarily; yet it will be found that they are in close relation to the more individual symbolism which was revealed to us by the association method, in which many ordinary images are sometimes found to be capable of a general symbolic interpretation. Let us take the instance of a dream about a dog. The associated ideas will teach us in what light we must regard this image. The dreamer may remember a dog he has seen the day before in the street, and this will give him occasion to talk about the lady who was walking with the dog, and who plays an important part in his emotional life, though he refuses to admit it. In this case the dog is not properly a symbol, but an indication or a help to memory.

There are other cases in which someone dreaming of a dog is reminded of a particular dog, but goes no further than that. For instance, he may recall various characteristic details of a dog, which he used to possess. He will tell how his dog was in the habit of barking very loudly at cats and pretending to be very courageous, yet as soon as a cat began to show anger, would walk past as if it did not see it. This may lead the dreamer to realise, however unwillingly, some of his own character-traits. In this case too the dog cannot be regarded as a symbol; but it might be said that this particular dog was a simile of some special characteristics.

Lastly, it may happen that the dreamer declares that no associated ideas occur to him. Sometimes this is caused by his involuntary repression of unpleasant associations. But he may also say: "Whatever I might think about a dog, could not be of any importance." If all the same we insist, the dreamer may respond by mentioning some well-known characteristics of dogs, such as faithfulness or watchfulness. If this idea can be brought into relation with the rest of the dream, it may very well be found to be consistent with the dream's meaning. In this case the dog will be used as a symbol, which is fairly widely accepted.

The above instances of interpretation, however incomplete, will serve to show how the relation between dream-images and associated thoughts may vary in value. When the interpretation of the dream symbols depends entirely on the dreamer's associated thoughts, we might talk of *individual* symbolism as opposed to *general* symbolism, in which the images possess some generally accepted symbolic meaning. In general symbolism the interpretation or translation may often seem somewhat strange and far-fetched to the dreamer, whereas in individual symbolism he will understand and accept the meaning quite readily. Freud assumes that general symbols, which need to be translated nowadays, used to be easily understood by everyone in the past. He writes (XV, p. 181) : "We seem to have come upon an ancient form of expression, which, except for a few fragments here and there, appears to have vanished from our knowledge." Thus it would seem as if traces of this ancient form of expression of the human mind may be found in dreams, and this is not to be wondered at when we remember that all our thoughts and expressions in dreams are on a lower level than in our waking life. All kinds of curious combinations of thought, which our critical conscious mind would not permit, occur quite freely in our dreams. I have not space to describe fully the peculiar laws that regulate the unconscious thinking and emotional life ; it is full of a variety of forms of thought and of feeling which belong mainly to primitive man, and which the modern mind is supposed to have outgrown. The study of dreams has opened a wide field of highly interesting and complicated problems, which many scientists will have to work at before they can be completely solved.

I hope that the above somewhat superficial descriptions of dream-symbols will suffice to show how difficult and lengthy any dream-analysis must necessarily be. It should only be undertaken by those who have studied the subject profoundly, for amateurishness may easily cause very serious mistakes. Some modern writers are apt to give the impression that the analysis of dreams chiefly consists in guessing intuitively at the meaning of dream-images. I must earnestly warn the reader against believing this to be true. No doubt we can sometimes interpret a dream without the dreamer providing any associated material ; but we can only arrive at a successful interpretation if we have a thorough knowledge of dream-problems in general, and of the dreamer's character and circumstances in particular. Even then the dreamer's own introspection will finally have to decide whether the interpretation is the right one.

We will now return to our original question : can we assume the existence of repressed unconscious processes in a normal person ; and if so, are these of the same nature as those that are the cause of hysterical symptoms ? Freud undoubtedly, from his study of dreams and small disturbances in conscious life, came to the conclusion that repressed unconscious processes are at work in a normal individual ; and this seems plausible enough to anyone who remembers that our modern culture requires the suppression of much that is natural. If we were always obliged to deal consciously with what we must repress, our mental life would be wholly occupied with this, and so it is a good thing that we gradually learn to allow our expressions to flow automatically along certain channels. Some people succeed so well in suppressing what is useless to them, that they are never aware of this process; and they would reject as incredible the idea that they too possessed an unconscious emotional background. Therefore repression in itself is rather a condition of health than a morbid symptom. The significant characteristic of abnormal people is that their repression is not complete, and that these hidden forces are not kept down sufficiently, but keep cropping up and giving rise to disturbances. They suffer from having tried to repress more than they were capable of. This may be due to one of two causes: either they have had to deal with unuseable emotions that are more numerous and strong than with normal people, or else they may have aimed at repressing the emotions which the normal man would naturally express. There are thus two types of neurotics; first those who possess a very difficult and unharmonious disposition, containing many useless and contradictory elements; secondly those who possess a more normal disposition, but make excessive demands upon it, in order to fulfil which, they have to repress every unsuitable element in their nature. This naturally leads us to the question whether the content of the unconscious is the same in the healthy mind as in the morbid. We saw that Freud found that the content of the unconscious in hysterical patients was based chiefly on sexuality in its widest sense. Is this also the case with the unconscious of normal people? After reading Freud we come to the conclusion that in his opinion, though sexuality plays an important part in the normal unconscious life, it must not be supposed to be the only factor. There are many other tendencies, besides sexuality, which are often repressed, such as ambition, cupidity, malice, cruelty; and we find instances of the repression of these emotions in the dreams quoted by Freud. It is all the same unnecessary for me to demonstrate that there is a great deal of repressed sexuality in many healthy people, as they are strongly influenced by the fear of social conventions. If we are accustomed to introspection, and are honest enough to acknowledge the character of the thoughts and emotions which we sometimes detect in ourselves, we may discover many surprising qualities in human nature. But unfortunately only few people nowadays take pains to discover the truth about themselves, and this is probably one of the reasons why Freud's theories about the unconscious have met with so much opposition. He is frequently attacked for laying too much stress on the sexual impulses in the emotional life. This reproach is probably founded on a misunderstanding of the term sexuality. He includes under this term all the feelings and expressions which are related to the development of the sexual emotions. This is contrary to ordinary usage and may cause some confusion, but anyone acquainted with the course of Freud's studies will easily understand and accept his terminology. I shall try to avoid the use of such terms as much as possible, as they are often misunderstood by those who have hitherto used them in a somewhat different sense. All the same according to the latest theories the sexual impulses, in the narrowest sense, are of great psychological importance. Miss M. K. Bradby has illustrated, by an interesting comparison, the general repugnance aroused by Freud's theory that many psychical manifestations are derivations of the sexual instinct, though not commonly thought to be so (V, p. 46).

" Let us suppose that instead of a sexual motive he had put his finger upon an ' acquisitive ' motive, which is in fact no less universal. Man is by nature acquisitive, desirous of acquiring and of possessing for himself every object which takes his fancy or promises to satisfy his desires. So far we all agree, but our imaginary Freud would go on to say that in consequence of this strong and innate instinct of man, we were all thieves in will if not in deed. He would point to the scrupulosity of strictly honest people as a proof of their hidden desire to steal, and he would convict us of refraining from theft, not out of any natural goodness, but because we were afraid of public opinion, afraid of the concrete penalties of the human law or of the magical penalties of the divine. He might work out his theory by analysing the dreams of dishonest people, show exactly how it was that they came to steal, and classify the various forms of stealing prevalent, recognised and unrecognised. Now to the average middle-class person, though he might not be disposed to agree, there would be nothing especially revolting in all this, because the accusation does not ' touch him on the raw.' He would think Freud was one-sided, but he would be prepared to treat his views with respect and to give him credit for taking a scientific and not a morbid interest in his special subject. The lady however who owes her washerwoman, the man who does not pay his debts, might dislike being convicted of a particularly mean form of stealing, and if deliberately paying less for a thing than one knew it was worth were included under the heading, still more people might feel indignant at the charge. Very poor people would be touched more nearly. When you are often hungry and cold because you are poor, it is difficult not to feel bitterly envious of less honest people who 'help themselves' in safe ways, and difficult not to be 'touchy' on the point of one's own honesty. How many people who are honest have thought the subject out and know just why they are honest, and why they would urge a poor man to go to the workhouse rather than to steal?

"But the case would be different if the struggle to be honest were an absorbing difficulty in the background of most people's minds, if secret thieving in various forms were universal, and if many people's lives were marred, and to a greater or lesser extent rendered miserable, because of the extreme or heroic measures they took to check their own thieving propensities. To treat the subject then in a cold, calm, detached and scientific manner would seem an outrage against humanity. We should all be up in arms against a theory which assumed us to be as bad as we really are, and worse, whatever might be the motives of its adherents. Nevertheless, we should be mistaken, because in the long run any light from whatever quarter thrown upon the origin and nature of dishonesty helps men to become honest in will and deed."

The above quotation indicates the peculiar position of the sexual impulse among all our other impulses, for it is the only one that is systematically repressed from early youth upwards, without any regard to possible injury to the whole emotional life. Recent scientific investigations have clearly proved, what was known for a long time by all good pedagogues, that sexual expressions are most intimately connected with all possible forms of love, so that the total repression of sexuality may easily give rise to disturbances of the more delicate emotions, such as a lack of balance or emotional dishonesty. Repression is then substituted for self-control. Children are usually taught to dissimulate very early, and instead of being given the right sort of instruction and guidance, are met with reproof and punishment, which they do not understand. Very few parents are sufficiently unprejudiced on this subject to give their children the help they need. The result is that the child often suffers from inner conflict, or is led into bad habits, and for a long time may secretly cling to the wrong forms of emotional expression. The same difficulty is met with in later life. It is considered wrong or indecent to talk about sexual problems and difficulties. One may only hint at them in a jocular way; any serious treatment is forbidden. The fact that a man has found an apparently satisfactory form of self-expression, such as marriage, is by no means a guarantee that he has succeeded in bringing harmony into his emotional expressions.

Imperfections in the early development of the emotions often vindicate themselves in later life. No one who is convinced of this will find any difficulty in accepting Freud's theory that the chief source of a great many nervous diseases is to be found in disturbances of the sexual life in all its ramifications, caused by repression of sexual problems. These delicate and subtle questions are apt to be treated in a coarse and summary way in our modern social life, without paying any heed to the intricacies of emotional development.

A simple-minded or well-balanced nature will suffer less mental disturbance from this summary and conventional attitude than one more delicate or complicated. The former type will more easily find a way out, and will in general conform to conventional ideals only in so far as they do not interfere with the satisfaction of his desires. But the more complicated character will take these conventional ideals much more seriously, because he hopes to find in them the solution of his inner conflict. People of this kind often suffer from more or less serious neurotic symptoms as a result of their failure to live up to ideals which they have really misunderstood. It is sometimes said that Freud would advise such persons to allow unrestrained liberty to all their instincts as a cure; but he is evidently far too clever a psychologist ever to have made such statements. Rather he aims at bringing these problems into the consciousness of his patients, so as to enable them to find a new harmony between their emotions. This advice is by no means intended to do away with all restraint. Nevertheless there is a good deal to be said against the ordinary ideals of our time, to which otherwise these patients would have conformed.

I must now return to the two determining factors of a neurosis due to repression, which I described above as firstly a difficult and unharmonious disposition, and secondly as the tendency to repress too much. In most cases these two factors will be found to co-operate, though in various proportions; and this is most clearly seen in sexual matters. In the following chapter we shall describe how, as a result of a difficult disposition, of unfavourable circumstances, or of an injudicious education, the sexual emotions may be led into the wrong channels; and we shall also show the bad influence this may have on the other emotions. The wrong forms of expression which will then arise, will be all the more readily repressed, if the patient is governed by high ideals and delicately developed emotions; but sometimes these ideals are so exaggerated that all sexual expression is regarded as inferior and discreditable, and the patient will then tend to adopt the same attitude to the greater part of his other emotions. In such a case we must consider that the neurotic symptoms are due not to the nature of the repressed material, but rather to a mistaken ideal, and the treatment will therefore aim in the first place at criticising this ideal. Some psychologists, especially Adler of Vienna, consider this to be the exclusive cause of most neuroses (I). According to him the nature of the neurotic disposition is a childish feeling of inferiority, which causes in the patient a reaction, which takes the form of an obstinate wish to make his personality felt, and a desire for power combined with the pursuit of high and unattainable ideals. Freud agrees with this; but his point of view seems to me to be somewhat wider. He too regards the exaggerated ego-ideal as the cause of disturbances (XIII, p. 17); but he thinks that these may also arise as the result of repression of unconscious desires by this ego-ideal, which is as it were the representative of our conscious personality, and thus assumes the power of repression. In so far as the morbid symptoms are an expression of the compromise between the repressed elements and the repressing power, we are no doubt right in considering the exaggerated ego-ideal as the cause of these symptoms; but it seems to me that Adler's theory is only justified in those cases where the ego-ideal is entirely predominant, and that in most other cases Freud's theory throws a better light on the complicated causes of neuroses.

The question may well be asked whether we must then reject our former beliefs, and consider it dangerous to strive after an ideal? Our answer must be that on the contrary a high ideal may provide a great support to the development of an individual, provided the ideal is in sufficient harmony with his natural disposition, and is the expression of its potentialities. But the ego-ideal may be a source of danger if he loses sight of the distance that divides him from his ideal, and is inclined to identify himself with it; he will then ignore his shortcomings, and satisfy himself with his good intentions, and he will ascribe virtues to himself which properly belong to his ideal. As he will expect his neighbours to recognise and appreciate these virtues, this will often lead to conflict, and he will be looked upon as arrogant and conceited. In such a case it is not necessary to destroy the ideal, so long as the individual can be made to understand the wrong use he was making of it.

It is clear that in most cases both the nature of the ideal, and the way it is used, might be improved, which implies that the ideal might well be pushed somewhat into the background, so as to avoid its insistent interference at every turn; thus room will be made for other expressions, such as affection, which shed a warmer and kindlier light on human life.

Cases may also occur when the conscious ideal is free from all strained exaggeration, and the suppression of an important part of the disposition is not due to the influence of this ideal, but to special difficulties inherent in the disposition itself. But if its nature is not essentially different from that of a normal person, the way towards sublimation can usually be found, as soon as a conscious effort is made in that direction and the suppression is removed.

If we look back upon the various psychological problems discussed above, it becomes clear that there is no very marked line separating the normal from the abnormal mind. The same contrast may be observed in normal people between the ego-ideal and the difficulties inherent in their character, although their ideal is usually a less strained conception, and their disposition more harmonious than is the case with the abnormal. Normal persons also suffer from unrecognised repressions, though the repression may be less thorough and recognition more easily attained than in abnormal cases In normal persons the unconscious is expressed in a less disturbing manner; but it may all the same be the source of some curious characteristics, of which they themselves are unaware. Almost every human being has these weak points in his character, which are sometimes of great and sometimes of little importance, but are nearly always better known to his family, friends and servants than to himself. Usually we learn more about anyone's unconscious life by these small weaknesses, than by his dreams or conscious disturbances. His whole emotional life is revealed rather by small occurrences and delicate shades of expression than by violent outbursts. Though sometimes it may be difficult to prove the existence of such unconscious qualities of the mind, we shall find that quite ordinary people usually know very well how to interpret these small weaknesses which they observe in someone with whom they have daily intercourse. The psycho-analytical method by which we search into the depths of the unconscious is by no means the only way to attain self-knowledge. Great men, through all the ages, have succeeded in gaining this self-knowledge, and developing themselves, by methods which everyone is free to use, and of which psycho-analysis is a somewhat more technical and systematic expansion. We can bring our hidden unconscious processes to the light of consciousness simply by observing our expressions, and our relations to other people, and by studying the way other people react to these expressions. We shall then begin to understand how our character is gradually modified by experience and circumstances, and we shall see the inter-relation between our past and present emotions, which are the outcome and expression of a similar impulse, however much they may have changed in the course of time. The actions and relationships of normal people depend upon the conditions and emotions of their childhood, and are chiefly explained by them, just as the morbid symptoms of a patient are caused by emotions and circumstances of childhood which prepared the way for the later neurotic reaction. The study of this problem belongs to the psychology of the emotions, which I shall treat in the next chapter.

CHAPTER III

THE DEVELOPMENT OF THE EMOTIONS

In this chapter I intend to give a short survey of Freud's work on the development of the emotions, which may be of greater interest to the general reader than the interpretation of dreams or the origin and character of neuroses. I shall assume that the methods which led Freud to formulate his theories are now sufficiently well known, and shall only be concerned here with the conclusions he reached after studying a great number of very intricate case-histories. It ought not to be demanded of Freud that these conclusions should be formulated in one complete system, because they depend principally upon his observations of his patients, and are thus continually being amplified. His theories also reveal their practical origin, by being mainly concerned with difficulties and disturbances which occur in various stages of the emotional development. Thus the chief conclusion to be drawn from his observations is that certain special difficulties in the emotional development may cause special disturbances in later life; and, vice versa, it may be inferred that the development of a certain kind of patient has been arrested by corresponding disturbances.

We have seen that we must assume a gradual transition between the normal and the abnormal; and that just as in abnormal persons the history of their symptoms can be traced to their development, so various characteristics of normal persons are connected with former circumstances and conflicts. Thus the difficulties met with in the emotional development may result according to the nature of their solution either in morbid symptoms or in mere character traits. This interesting connection was discovered by others before Freud. Some neuroses were known to reveal themselves as morbid exaggerations of certain types of character: but Freud has thrown a great deal of new light on the matter.

Emotional difficulties may appear quite early in childhood, and one of Freud's most striking discoveries is that the emotional experiences of childhood exercise a predominating influence upon later development. This is in clear contradiction to the prevailing opinion that human character is chiefly determined by heredity. But I must add that Freud does not entirely deny the importance of heredity, though he has severely criticised those who wish to explain everything by means of it.

It is clear that the emotions play an important part at a much earlier stage than reason. An infant not only expresses its emotions in an emphatic manner, but also makes use of such expression to attain satisfaction of its desires. We are so accustomed to connect these exhibitions of emotion in ourselves and others with reasoned conceptions, that some may doubt whether similar exhibitions in infants can be already termed emotional. The only satisfactory method of solving this question would be by introspection. If we could clearly recall the emotions of our infancy and our expression of them, we ought to be able to decide whether we then possessed emotions of the same nature as in later life. As this is impossible, we must employ another method, which we do in fact use every day in other cases: we must determine the character of the emotions from their expression. We then see that the mother clearly perceives the feelings expressed by the infant before it can talk clearly; and we find that the emotional life of the infant is closely connected with its physical needs, such as feeding, sleep, excretory acts and washing. The infant depends on others for the satisfaction of its emotional needs; but it has already discovered that a strong expression of discontent can bring about the satisfaction it desires. Thumb-sucking is also one of the ways by which some infants try to satisfy themselves. Probably this replaces the gratification of being fed. Later on other bodily sensations may come into play. It is probable that some children enjoy the sensation of tension caused by the holding back of stool or urine. They try to prolong this sensation as much as possible, and obstinately refuse to be trained in methodical habits which might interfere with these sensations. At this point the conflict caused by the suppression and control of natural impulses arises for the first time. The manner in which the infant reacts to such training, foreshadows certain important characteristics of its later life. It is worth while considering this question somewhat more closely.

Freud discovered early in his investigations that a relation existed between certain character traits and irregularities in the control of excretions during childhood (X, p. 132). These character traits are orderliness, parsimony and self-will. The sense of order includes physical neatness, accuracy and reliability. Parsimony may develop into miserliness, and self-will easily becomes obstinacy. In consequence of this discovery he assumed that these traits represented a later development of an earlier emotional conflict. Thus neatness and orderliness are a later reaction against an original childish tendency to oppose neat and orderly methods, and to find a certain satisfaction in bed-wetting. Obstinacy is the development of the child's tendency not to pay attention to its elders in such matters. Parsimony illustrates the connection between the desire to retain faeces and the desire to retain money, instances of which constantly occur in common speech and fairy-tales. It may throw light on this relation between precious gold and the most despised and disgusting of material objects, if we remember that the attitude of disgust towards excrement is not a natural one with most children. On the contrary they attach great interest to it, as it is associated with not unpleasant bodily sensations; and if not interfered with, they would often use it for moulding and smearing. Although parents and others may speedily teach them that it is objectionable and dirty to occupy themselves with excrements, yet on the other hand the importance of these things is thus impressed on their minds. The child is praised when it has done " its duty," and called good and clever. Thus for a long time this function is associated in its mind with important emotions, especially if it is accompanied by difficulties. These difficulties can have two origins: either a natural sensitiveness of the organs, owing to which the emotions are unduly stimulated by pleasant or unpleasant sensations; or else some malady of the organs in childhood which may make them over-sensitive, or specially direct the child's attention to them. The experience of children's doctors shows that children suffering from intestinal disease often grow up into discontented, irritable and melancholy human beings.

It should now be easy to answer certain questions which may well occur to students of Freud's theories. Even if it be agreed that there is this connection between excretory disturbances and certain character-traits, is it so certain, it might be asked, that these traits are caused by the child's taking such pleasure in retaining the faeces and depositing them according to its own choice? Is it not more likely that these childish traits reveal the inherited basis of its later character? In this case it might be possible to regard the whole childish episode as something accidental, without which its character would develop in just the same trend. It is no doubt true that if we attempt to trace back any human traits to their remotest origins, we shall find them expressed at a very early and simple stage, for the original disposition is always the same. At the same time when Freud deduces these psychical traits from some special physical peculiarity—in this case a natural hyper-sensitiveness of the anal mucous membrane—we certainly ought not to reject this conclusion because it seems unpleasant or materialistic. Experience must finally decide in such a case; and it would be interesting to investigate whether children, who originally have not shown any symptoms of this kind of hyper-sensitiveness, are found to develop these special character-traits after a chronic abdominal illness. Though Freud's theory that psychical traits are due to physical conditions may be incomplete yet his remarks about the way these traits change under the influence of environment, are of great value. The inter-relations between orderliness, parsimony and self-will, and the ways in which they express themselves, are no doubt very various, and depend chiefly on other character-traits. But this subject is too complicated to be fully treated here.

The emotions associated with passing water, are also sometimes of importance, because they may create other disturbances and peculiarities in the general emotional development. They are moreover in close relation to the later sexual emotions, which is understandable when we remember in what close proximity the sexual organs are to the organs of excretion. During strong tension of the bladder and at its evacuation, many children experience special sensations, which are akin to the feelings experienced during discharge of the sexual organs. Such children will find it difficult to abstain from the satisfaction of bed-wetting, although they are not clearly conscious of the reason. It may happen that such difficulties in childhood will recur again in the form of some disturbance at a later age.

We have seen that the emotional life of the small child, though it may seem simpler than the adult's, presents all possible varieties and degrees of emotion, which are chiefly expressed by the bodily functions. As the child develops, these functions increase in number, and so create new sources of emotion. It begins to move and to walk, and the noises it makes grow more and more full of meaning. In contrast with the first infantile period, which was much more passive and under the influence of the alimentary functions and everything connected with them, this second period might be described as the period of desire for movement, in which activity and passivity are found in opposition. This desire for movement leads to many opportunities of experiencing pain-sensations, which again may lead to emotions of anger or fear. The desire to possess and control becomes more and more evident at this stage. The emotions connected with the excretory functions are growing in importance, as the struggle to control these functions is now taking place.

The psychic life of the child is at this time being gradually co-ordinated. The process is accelerated, if not caused, by the beginnings of thought; while thought in its turn is strongly stimulated by the beginnings of speech. The result of this co-ordination is that sensations are experienced much more by the whole body as a unit, than by the separate organs. The child's attention is more concentrated upon its own body, and this contemplation and investigation is sometimes connected with strong emotions, which are naturally still much influenced by the organic sensations that used to be predominant. Here we see a process that frequently takes place in the emotional life, the gradual growth of new expressions of emotion from older ones. In this period of co-ordination the child's own body, and later on its ego, becomes the centre of the chief emotional satisfactions. The child not only finds satisfaction in looking at itself, in practising walking and other movements, and in performing various tricks, but it likes being looked at when undressed, or when it is performing its newly acquired movements. Sometimes it shows great sensitiveness to praise or blame, which either strengthen or oppose its emotions. Thus we see that the child's emotions are not exclusively connected with its bodily functions. Already some emotional relation exists with the outer world; and this relation is gradually developed in conjunction with the emotions that we have been describing, though it is only at a later stage that it becomes a guiding force in the emotional life.

At an early age the child becomes aware that the sensations caused by certain bodily functions are connected with a powerful beneficent intervening influence. The psychic life at the very beginning is probably too indeterminate for the child to make even a vague distinction between the ego and the non-ego, so that probably the mother is more or less identified with its own body. This will make it all the easier for the child at a later stage to transfer its pleasurable emotions to the mother, who seems to be so closely connected with them. At this early stage the nature of these emotions is determined entirely by bodily condition. The child experiences its mother almost exclusively as the one who gives satisfaction. Later on too this remains the prevailing point of view; but as soon as educational difficulties arise, the relation to the mother grows much more complicated, as she is often forced to refuse satisfaction. The child will then learn the importance of reading on the mother's face whether its emotional desires have a good or bad chance of being satisfied; and as soon as it has learnt that it can change its mother's face by expressing itself in various ways, it will try to influence events by these means. We have seen that being taught habits of cleanliness may cause complications in the child's emotional relations with its surroundings, and may produce a tendency to resist interference and to react with anger. Up to this point we have found that the influence of the outside world upon the child was only of importance in so far as it stimulated or opposed the emotions connected with its own body. It is only after its own ego has been discovered and its limits realised, that it becomes possible for the child to obtain a clear view of the outside world, or to conceive the existence of other egos besides itself, and understand their emotions and desires as contrasted with its own. Conversely the child is prepared for the realisation of its own ego by attempts to enter into the thoughts and feelings of other people, for example by imitating them. As soon as it realises this division between the ego and the non-ego, innumerable problems and difficulties arise in the child's life. It is true that it generally derives great satisfaction from this discovery of the ego, by which means alone it is able to become acquainted with the outer world, where it can gratify its desires. But these advantages go together with considerable disillusionment; for it is only now that the child perceives how much more dependent it is on external forces than on its own will and desires. No wonder that it does not reach a clear perception of this conflict at once, so that it is only after a long period of internal and external struggle that it can rightly understand the relation between the ego and the outer world. No wonder too that in the history of mankind, numerous more or less successful solutions of this problem have been formulated by religions and philosophies, and that many people in their emotional life never succeed in satisfactorily solving this conflict, which they became aware of for the first time when they were about three years old.

The most usual result of this inner change in the child is that it realises more clearly its own dependence upon its surroundings, and so tries to get into closer touch with them. Hence the child's environment is apt to have a preponderating influence on the further development of its emotional life. A child surrounded by loving care will tend to judge lightly of the difficulties it meets with when seeking to satisfy its emotional needs, and will be ready to put its trust in life. Another child that is treated roughly and brutally may easily be overpowered by a hopeless sense of incapacity to satisfy its needs, and will probably turn its longings towards its early state of ignorance, which was less painful. These two extremes are bridged by many transitional stages. Most children, when difficult demands are made of them, will be inclined at times to shut their eyes upon the whole outside world and its complications, and to concentrate on their own emotional needs alone, just as they used to do so much more easily in early days. Here we find a sharp contrast between the two principles which govern the psychic life, the " pleasure-principle " and the " reality-principle " (XII), and here too is the source of the life of the phantasy, which often begins to appear at this age, and is strongly influenced, in its form, by the child's newly acquired mental powers, though its emotional bias is much more determined by the previous stage of development. By this phantasy process the child is again enabled to find gratification of various desires; but whereas in a former stage this gratification was found more by purely physical means, the psychic life will now tend to gain the upper hand. All the same, when difficulties arise in the way of gratifying the emotional desires, the need of physical gratification may again come to the fore.

If circumstances are at all favourable, this period between the third and sixth year is chiefly marked by the new relationships formed by the child with its surroundings. And in the first place the relationship with the parents is of great importance, and may be of various kinds. At this age children often show a preference for one of the parents, and it is noteworthy that the difference of sex often influences their choice. Not only does the young son feel a strong attraction towards the mother, but he begins to look upon his father as a rival. This often finds expression in such sayings as, " I will marry my mother when I am grown-up," or, " Father had better go away on a journey, or to the war, and then I will look after mother." The child has only a vague notion of death. His only idea about it is that " dying " and " going away " are the same thing; and so the child may easily come to say that the father may as well die, and then he will marry his mother. Freud has named this the Oedipus-complex, from the Greek tragedy, in which Oedipus is driven by the Fates to kill his father and to marry his mother. Freud's theory that the great impression made by this tragedy is due to the fact that we have all felt similar desires at a certain stage of our life, has created much indignation and anxiety. A confusion has usually been made between two of Freud's theories, firstly that this Oedipus-complex may be of decisive importance in the emotional life of some people, especially neurotics, and secondly that everyone has felt similar emotions at some stage of his development. The possible disastrous results of the Oedipus-complex, which usually appear only at puberty, I shall deal with later. At present I will only point out that we should be misunderstanding Freud, if we applied this theory too strictly to any normal person. In his last book (XV, p. 381) he writes as follows: "What does direct observation of the child, at the time of the selection of its object, before the latent period, show us concerning the Oedipus-complex? One may easily see that the little man would like to have the mother all to himself, that he finds the presence of his father disturbing; he becomes irritated when the latter permits himself to show tenderness towards the mother, and expresses his satisfaction when the father is away or on a journey. Frequently he expresses his feelings directly in words, and promises the mother he will marry her. One may think this is very little in comparison with the deeds of Oedipus, but it is actually enough, for it is essentially the same thing. The observation is frequently clouded by the circumstance that the same child, on other occasions, gives evidence of great tenderness towards its father; this only means that such contradictory, or rather *ambivalent* emotional attitudes as would lead to a conflict in the case of an adult, readily take their place side by side in a child, just as later on they permanently exist in the unconscious. Someone might object that the behaviour of the child springs from egoistic motives, and does not justify the hypothesis of an erotic complex. The mother provides for all the necessities of the child, and it is therefore to the child's advantage that she should trouble herself for no one else. This is true ; but it will soon be clear that in this, as in similar situations, the egoistic interest merely offers the opportunity which the erotic impulse seizes upon. If the child shows the most undisguised sexual curiosity about his mother, if he wants to sleep with her at night, and insists upon being present while she is dressing, or even tries in his childish way to play the seducer, as the mother can often clearly perceive, and afterwards laughingly relates, it is undoubtedly due to the erotic nature of the attachment to his mother. We must not forget that the mother shows the same care for her little daughter without producing the same effect, and that the father often vies with her in care for the boy without being able to win the same importance in his eyes as the mother does. In short, it is clear that the factor of sex preference cannot be eliminated from the situation by any kind of criticism."

It is clear that Freud has used the term Oedipus-complex more in order to indicate the nature of the emotions, than to imply the presence of a tragic conflict. In the case of a little girl, the emotional relation is somewhat of the same nature. Her egoistic motives do not point in the same direction as her erotic ones, for she sees it is to her interest to maintain good relations with her mother, as she is dependent on her care, while the father is mostly absent. Tenderness and caresses from the mother will no doubt also bring about greater intimacy between mother and daughter. Yet it constantly happens, especially when there are several daughters in the family, that the attraction between father and daughter appears quite early, and often coincides with a certain jealousy of the mother by the daughter. The parents themselves often influence this emotional complex, because they also may unconsciously be affected by the difference of sex.

We must be on our guard against judging the child's emotional life according to adult standards, because the emotions at this early stage have a peculiar character of their own. Our present knowledge shows us that our unconscious life is closely related to the infantile emotions, and this helps us towards a better understanding of their peculiar character. In a child contradictory emotions can exist side by side much more easily than in an adult. A child can show great affection and tenderness for someone who the next moment will arouse its fury and rage. Greed and generosity can alternate very rapidly. Little children generally exhibit all kinds of primitive emotions. They take great pleasure in breaking things to pieces and in causing pain, but these emotions are usually quickly superseded by others. The less kindly emotions are especially shown towards brothers and sisters. When a child hears that the stork has brought another little brother or sister, its feelings will be very mixed. It will soon perceive that the new arrival claims most of the parent's interest and care, and that it will have to be satisfied with less. Jung relates the instance of a girl of four years, who was going to have a little brother (XXIII, p. 9). The father put the child on his knee and asked, "What would you say if you were to get a little brother to-night?" "Then I would kill it," was the immediate answer. Of course we must not lay too much stress on the word

" kill," because the child had no clear conception of what it meant ; all the same it expressed her feelings clearly enough.

When we realise of what enormous importance the arrival in the family of a new child can be to an older one, and how fundamentally it may transform its emotional life, we shall easily believe that small children begin quite early to be interested in the question of where babies come from. We may at first doubt the intensity of this curiosity, because most children do not show it except by a few questions, and seem to be easily satisfied with the ordinary stories about storks and cabbages. But investigations have revealed that the parents' reticence may often have far-reaching results of which they have no idea. In the first place children often notice that they are given an evasive answer, and the slight embarrassment of the parent at their questions gives them the feeling that some secret or other is being hidden from them. The curious result is that they do not mention the subject any more because they do not quite trust the parent's information, or, if they do continue their questions, they do so in such a roundabout way that they are often misunderstood. Another result of the unsatisfying answer may be that the child's attention is now more drawn to the problem, which might otherwise have been put aside. The child often sees and hears much more than the parents imagine, and so may easily find a starting point for speculation ; but as some important facts nearly always remain hidden, the result of all this vague searching will be quite fantastic. An observant child may easily deduce the fact that the infant comes out of the mother's body, but it is more difficult to find out exactly how. Judging from experience of its own body, the child naturally sees a connection with its excrements, which are also produced from its body. Thus the idea arises that the infant leaves the body by the anus. In this way the child may come to imagine that it can produce an infant itself. A little precocious boy of three years old had been told by his parents that a new baby would arrive in a couple of months. At a children's party he said to his hostess, pointing to his abdomen, " I have a baby in my tummy. Listen ! you can hear him grumbling. He is coming out to-morrow."

This knowledge leads to new questions as to how the baby gets into the mother's abdomen, and also as to what part the father plays. As the connection between food and excretion is known, the idea may arise that the origin of the baby is to be found in something the mother has eaten. Or there may be other theories, as for instance that the baby is produced by means of an operation ; or else fantastic ideas connected with death may appear. The following dialogue took place between a little girl of three years old and her grandmother (XXIII, p. 8).

Anna. " Grandmother, why are your eyes so wrinkled ? "

Grandmother. " Because I am so old."

Anna. " I know ; but then you will grow young again."

Grandmother. " No ; for, you know, I shall grow older and older until I die."

Anna. " And then ? "

Grandmother. " Then I shall become an Angel."

Anna. " But then you will be turned into a little child again ? "

A year later, after the birth of a little brother, this same child whispered anxiously and mistrustfully into its mother's ear, " Are you sure you won't die now ? "

These birth theories probably play this important rôle in the child's life, because they are so closely connected with the physical images and sensations which predominate at this period. Sexual feelings may have something to do with it also, though we must be on our guard against identifying this kind of sexual expression with that of later life. The emotions are still but little differentiated : they are still in a closely-knit tangle, out of which later on definite shapes will arise. Two facts which help to emphasise the connection between the excretory functions and vague sexual sensations, are first the close local connection between the organs, and secondly the atmosphere of secrecy and of the forbidden which surrounds them both. Also disturbances in the excretory organs may cause a stimulus leading to an early habit of masturbation.

The importance which children attach to their physical sensations is clearly revealed in their relations to others. They often show curiosity as to the bodily functions of parents or equals, and are greatly interested in watching other people's excretory functions. If they are left at all free, they will find expression for these feelings in many of their games, such as playing at being a doctor, or " keeping house," the details of which will show the importance to them of physical intimacy. Even falling in love with a playfellow, or a brother or sister, may occur in this early stage of budding erotic sensations.

Now that we know how deep is the influence of the early stages of emotional expression upon later life, we can easily understand the very great importance of the child's position in the sequence of his brothers and sisters. With an only child the relation to the parents will be preponderant, while in a large family this may be compensated for by other relations. Thus the later social feelings of an only child will be strongly influenced by its feelings towards its parents. Especially if such a child has been spoilt, it will retain for a long time the impression that the gratification of its desires can be easily obtained. It is used to having everyone at its beck and call and ministering to its needs. This may grow into such a habit, that the child will feel it as a great injustice in later life, if it does not continue to form the centre of its surroundings.

When we consider the relations of the eldest child in the family, we must not forget that it once occupied the favoured position of an only child, and that at a certain moment it was dispossessed. Of course it is important to know at what age the successor appeared, because the effect on the child may be much more complicated when it is already three or four years old, than when it is younger. But even where the difference of age is only slight, the effects of this dispossession are felt deeply enough to give rise to complicated reactions. When the older child feels that it receives less affection and care from the mother, it may seek for compensation from the father, or from someone else in its surroundings, who in turn will then become the centre of the child's emotional life. If it does not succeed in finding such compensation, an emotional regression may occur, and the child will then centre its emotional life upon itself, just as it used to do unconsciously at the time of its physical interest in itself But now more complicated results arise. The child will appear to attach less importance to care and affection of which it now feels the lack, and will pretend to have outgrown those needs. A boy especially will then make an effort to appear brave and grown-up ; he will emphasise all the attainments in which he is superior to his younger brother or sister, and this feeling of superiority will be a great consolation. An elder sister will tend to become more motherly with the younger ones. Altogether this change in the child's life may be a strong stimulus to the intellectual and phantasy-life, and may also have a far-reaching influence on the later character. The desire of the eldest to be independent and to dominate over the younger, will often arise from this first conflict.

The position of the youngest child has also its peculiarities. It enjoys the advantage of not being dispossessed of its rights by a younger successor. On this point the case is somewhat similar to that of the only child. It does in fact sometimes get spoilt, but its joys are not unadulterated. The fate of Joseph, who was ill-treated by his brothers, and finally sold as a slave, is an apposite case. The youngest has to defend the privileges showered on him by the parents against the attacks of his older brothers and sisters. He will feel that special favours are due to him, and at the same time may be in fear of subjection, which may give rise to angry feelings towards these elders, and to a desire to pay them out and be their master. In later life this may result in a feeling of rancour towards equals, side by side with love and respect towards those in high authority.

It might be thought that the position of the middle child was of a less definite type, and would have less far-reaching results. This is certainly not the case (XIX). One of the strongest influences is the uncertainty of its position. Sometimes it is included with the elder ones, sometimes with the younger, and it has less privileges than either the youngest or the eldest. As soon as it has obtained some privilege, it may have to be given up to the younger ones. The eldest or the youngest are often chosen out for a special treat; the middle child will always have to share it with one of the others. The eldest will treat the middle child as inferior, and the youngest will feel itself its equal. Hence often a certain bitterness, and a feeling of enmity both towards older or younger brothers or sisters. Sometimes it feels out of touch with them, and then withdraws into its ego, or seeks to find some satisfying relations outside its own family circle. Very often this may lead to the child's making its way more easily later on into society, as it is accustomed to make less demands than the others. But it may also give rise to a feeling of uncertainty and of being pushed into the background. The position of the middle child is most difficult when it is of the same sex as the older and younger. A girl coming between two boys may develop the typical feminine traits of "child wife" towards the older, and of "little mother" towards the younger. A boy between two girls will be sure to come to the front by means of his male characteristics.

When once the connection between these juvenile

circumstances and later character-traits has been understood, it is astonishing how constantly we come across illustrations. There are two reasons why this influence on the later development is so powerful, (*a*) because the influence described above, such as the relations to parents, brothers and sisters, is spread over a long period; and (*b*) because the child's mind is extremely sensitive to strong impressions, and is like wax in its plasticity at this early period. In some cases it is evident that a single event in childhood has influenced the whole of later life. The importance of such an event is due not only to the strong emotion aroused by it, but to the fact that these emotions are closely connected with fundamental impulses. We constantly find that an event during this plastic period has determined the trend of sexual expression for the rest of life. With some people sexual gratification is dependent upon unusual circumstances. Such deviations of the sexual instinct are called perversities. It used to be generally accepted that such perversities were the outcome of an inherited bias. Later investigations have proved that in most cases such abnormality was determined by some event in early childhood, when the sexual impulse was prematurely over-stimulated, either through sexual temptation by adults or older children, or through a sexual scene which the child may involuntarily have witnessed. I have treated a patient who as a child had been sexually excited by an adult's foot, with the result that later in life his sexual feelings were unusually roused by a special kind of foot. Most parents consider a child between two and four years old to be much more innocent than it really is, and so it often happens that children of that age continue to share their parents' bedroom, and thus see and hear things which they had better not. In this way feelings are aroused, especially in the case of nervous or over-sensitive children, which if their development had been normal, would have remained correlated with other emotions, until the later stage of normal and independent expression had been reached. Such a precociously aroused sexual emotion is not always easy to recognise as such. In the first place the form it takes is vague, and so the child is not clearly conscious of it, and the emotion often finds an outlet in anxiety or fear; also the child feels, often quite early in life, that it has done something that is forbidden, or witnessed what it was not meant to know; and the consequent emotional conflict forces it to banish such unpermitted experiences from its consciousness, that is to say to repress them. Hence inner conflicts, caused by external events, may produce later on great disturbances in the emotions, neurosis, and even insanity. The intensity of the early emotional life, though of great importance, is naturally not the only factor that determines further development. Freud has never maintained that all such early conflicts must irrevocably result in insanity, to which a great many more factors would have to contribute.

One of the most important events which may leave a lasting impression on the child's life, is the death of a near relation. The influence of such an event varies according to whether affection is felt for the deceased, or whether death removes a rival in the family's affections, so that a disturbance in emotional gratification is cleared away. In the first case the deprivation of affection may lead the child to seek consolation and compensation from someone else.

But very often this may not succeed, or only insufficiently; and then a curious phenomenon may appear, which we constantly meet with in later disturbances of emotional gratification: I mean regression, or a return to infantile expression. In the primary stage of its development, the child obtains expression for its love-emotions through its own mind or body. Lack of affection will drive the child back into this early stage. It will become self-centred; phantasy will supply the means to satisfy its needs, and its attention may again be drawn to various physical sensations which may help to supply some gratification. A small child generally has a yearning hunger for love, which is partly due to its sense of weakness and dependence. If it finds no satisfaction for this hunger, it may retreat into its own little world, and retain the impression of the callousness and enmity of the outer world for the rest of its life. Lack of love may also cause a reaction in the child, who may become sullen and cruel, as if it wished to prove to itself that all this need of affection is senseless, and that to be a victim and to victimise others is merely human destiny. If such children do not come into timely contact with people who understand their condition and needs, they will run great risk of growing up with spoilt and perverted emotions.

When a rival in affection is removed by death, the difficulties are of a very different kind. If the rival were only thought of as such, the consequences would be fairly simple. The circumstances that lead to spoiling, as in the case of an only child, would merely become more frequent. But it is not always so simple. We have seen that a child can experience contradictory emotions at the same time. Usually it will have also felt affectionate and friendly feelings towards its rival. When feelings of hatred and rivalry have been gratified, the child will not only become more clearly conscious of its opposite feelings, but it may become aware of the contradiction for the first time, and this often arouses a sense of guilt. When they have been gratified, it will think of its angry feelings as being bad, and a tragic feeling of remorse may be combined with grief for the loss of a dead parent or brother or sister. In this connection we sometimes find a peculiar characteristic that is more clearly marked in some children than in others. This is what Freud has called " the belief in the omnipotence of thought," which means that the child believes that its mere wishes are followed by immediate results in the external world. We find the same conviction prevailing in savages, who urge their chief to produce the wished-for rain by mere thinking, or ask the " medicine man " to bring illness upon their enemy by some incantation. Such analogies between the psychology of children and primitive people are constantly to be met with, and they are the foundation of many fruitful investigations by Freud and his followers. Space forbids me to treat them more fully; but we may assume that the child ascribes great power to its thoughts, and thus often feels specially responsible when the desired result seems to be obtained. The remorse for its earlier feelings and desires may find expression in exaggerated grief and display of affection for the dead rival, and may indeed have a lasting influence, which will chiefly take the form of a suspicious attitude towards its own emotions, manifested by over-anxiety, uncertainty and an exaggerated conscientiousness. A child often seems to be much altered by such an event. The desire for affection, which might be more easily gratified after the removal of the rival, is now disturbed by the feeling of guilt with which it remains associated. As with other emotional conflicts, we find that the problem is made more difficult, if not impossible, to solve, by its remaining in the regions of the unconscious or half-conscious. The struggle cannot be fought out, but remains in the background as a threatening influence affecting and disturbing all kinds of conscious processes.

Physical illness is of great importance among the many circumstances which may influence the child's emotional life. A child that has suffered from a long illness, is put back as a consequence into an earlier stage of its development. Everyone pets it and is at its beck and call; it is the centre of its surroundings, and shut off from the stimuli of the outer world, while its attention is strongly drawn towards its own ailing body and its own emotional life. Feelings of affection are pushed into the background by the importance of the ego. We find here some resemblance to the case of the child who has been spoilt, or else driven back into its own emotional life by lack of affection. But in the spoilt child the love of its parents still remains an influential factor; and the mind of the child in need of affection will be centred on its mental functions and activities more than is the case with the invalid, whose attention will be almost wholly occupied with the physical and passive side. So we need not wonder that a lengthy illness in this plastic period of youth should have a far-reaching influence on the later character. The emotions often retain their infantile mode of expression, and so their full development is hampered.

This primary stage is of great importance from the point of view of the later emotional life, because the mental functions, which alone enable the child to adapt itself to the outer world, are hardly yet developed, and so the inner impulses will have to find a simpler outlet of expression, which will be determined by the child's bodily condition and its surroundings. The conditions of the body will tend to control the first infantile period, while the influence of environment will predominate between the third and sixth year. This first period of bodily emotions up to the third year, can be divided into three sub-divisions:—(1) when the alimentary functions are of most importance, (2) when activity begins, and the struggle to learn habits of cleanliness takes place, (3) when the various physical emotions are being co-ordinated, and the consciousness of the ego and of the individual body is awakening. Freud combines the two first periods under the name of *auto-erotic* period (XI, p. 45), because the emotions are of a sensual kind and are connected with the body. He gives the name of *Narcissistic period* (XIII) to the time when the body as a whole forms the centre of the child's interest. This name is borrowed from the youth Narcissus, who according to Greek mythology fell in love with himself, and never grew tired of contemplating his own image mirrored in the water.

The transition from the Narcissistic period to the period when the emotions are directed outwards and grow into the so-called objective emotions (object-libido), is marked by the discovery of the ego and the non-ego. The reaction to this discovery creates in the child a feeling of dependence on the outer world, and makes him desire to be in closer relationship with it. We have already seen how strong an influence the circumstances of the child's life at this age may have on its emotional development, and how special events at this period may for ever determine the later character.

A disturbance, which develops in later life in consequence of abnormal conditions in early childhood, has been given the name of *fixation* by Freud. He wishes to indicate by this term, that a child's desire for gratification may be so influenced by circumstances, as to remain fixed in its earliest form of expression. The cause may be some physical peculiarity, such as pleasurable sensations during defaecation, or the fact that the child was spoilt by its parents. Other circumstances, such as illness or loss of affection, may have an indirect influence, by inducing the child to seek satisfaction in its phantasy life. But the result will always be a fixation of the gratification idea. Such fixation may hamper the normal development of the emotional life in two ways, by retardation and by regression. It is an instance of retardation when a sense of gratification remains connected with bed-wetting instead of being transferred to the sexual functions; or when a boy's emotions continue to be centred upon his mother during his whole life. But we should call it regression when a child, who has been clean for some time, falls back into old habits, because it has met with punishment or resistance when it was seeking for new forms of expression; or when a man, meeting with difficulties in his married life, re-directs the whole of his emotional life towards his mother. We find retardation and regression expressed in many varied forms. It is an instance of regression when a man comes to blows with another because he is at a loss for an argument. The sexual life, in its widest sense, is specially subject to similar disturbances. We have seen the importance of early childhood in this connection, because during that time the emotions are most rapidly transformed and developed.

After the sixth year the child has passed through most of its *Sturm-und-Drang* period. The emotional life has now become co-ordinated into a group of expressions, out of which it continues to develop as best it may, if no further disturbances take place. As mental power increases, and under the influence of the outer world in the form of school-life, sensitiveness will decrease. Reason will enable the child to work off its emotional tension, while at school it will find it easier freely to select and modify its relations with others. The difficulties experienced by the child at this stage are usually a weak reflection of those belonging to an earlier period. But in the case of the only child, it is now that it becomes aware of life's difficulties for the first time. School-life has also the effect of once more emphasising the emotions connected with the ego. Praise and punishment will tend to centre the child's attention upon itself.

Having passed through these years, which Freud calls the *latency-period*, the emotional life regains its predominating influence at *puberty* (XI). The general equilibrium, hitherto fairly well maintained, will now be upset, and many years will often elapse before a satisfactory readjustment is found. What is the real nature of the process that goes on during this period? It has been defined as the birth and development of the sexual emotions; but this explanation does not seem entirely satisfactory. Freud has proved that sexual emotions are experienced in early childhood, though in a less definite form, so that it would be a mistake to say that they appear now for the first time, which would also conflict with our knowledge that emotions nearly always arise out of earlier related emotions. Freud holds that the essence of puberty consists in these two changes: (1) vague sexual emotions now begin to centre themselves upon the sexual organs, and are thus directed towards a more definite object; (2) the impulse arises to focus all love and admiration upon one ideal object, which in return can gratify all the higher emotions. Both changes have very different results, and vary much in importance in different individuals.

The sensations connected with the sexual organs will tend to make the child more conscious of the difference of sex, and its attention will be drawn to other bodily sensations, which had been pushed into the background during the latency period. The phantasy life may now become more occupied with the products of an earlier stage. In any case both the physical and phantasy life will be increasingly centred round the sexual organs.

The influence of sexual maturity on the psychic life is manifested in quite a different way. The tendency to idealise, to find an object of admiration, is in contrast to the love-emotions of the former period; for now the object is usually sought for outside the family circle. This is a new departure, for it implies separation from the home, which will in the end lead to an independent position. But the loosening of these ties is not always easily accomplished. For a long time the father and mother have been the centre of the child's predominating emotions; and this fact often has an influence on the choice of a new person to idealise, when this loosening process takes place. The admiration and love of a boy is often directed towards a much older woman, and the young girl will often feel more attracted by older men than by her contemporaries.

Much light will be thrown on this matter if we perceive the connection between these two important changes during the puberty period. The search for an ideal object of love, and the direction of attention outside the family circle, are both due to the physical change which concentrates all erotic emotions upon the sexual organs. During the latency-period, the control of the bodily functions and the suppression of disturbing emotions has become fairly complete: the child has absorbed all sorts of current opinions about good and bad, about what is allowed and not allowed, until they have become a second nature. The superfluous part of the emotions has been suppressed, and the remainder is now mainly centred on the parents, of whom one is sometimes selected as the favourite. Though these emotions are sometimes of a vaguely erotic nature, they do not create a disturbing element among the other emotions with which they are closely combined. When a child happens to exercise its fantasy upon sexual matters, it will naturally include its parents in this connection. But when at puberty the vaguely erotic emotions are condensed into the sexual, in the narrow sense of the word, they will then appear to be in sharp contrast with the emotions the child feels for its parents, and also with everything it has learnt to regard as good and pure. The internal conflict which then follows may be solved in three ways. (1) The emotions may all remain associated together, yet be gradually detached from the parents, and directed towards some object, with whom sexual relations are not forbidden. (2) In some cases, children will find it very difficult to accomplish this process of detachment in an easy and gradual way ; consequently the irreconcilable emotions will be torn asunder, and the emotional life will become divided on the one side into high ideals and pure love, without any sexual element, and on the other into sensual impulses that are considered reprehensible, and connected with people of low origin, and are often gratified by masturbation. An example of such a solution is the young man who, having a sentimental adoration for his mother, thinks of woman as a being too sacred to be defiled by marriage, yet who at the same time gratifies his passions by short and superficial sexual relations. (3) In the third case the emotions are not detached from the parents, nor are they torn asunder and partially directed towards a new object. The difficulty created by these irreconcilable emotions is hidden away, and anything to do with sexual or useless emotions is promptly driven out of the conscious life. This will often require a strong effort of will, and the result will be that the problem seems to have disappeared. Such people appear to lack all sexual emotions, and the equilibrium of the latency-period seems to be continuous. But we have seen that such people are likely to suffer from hysterical or other morbid symptoms, because it is impossible to repress or divert these vitally important impulses without bad results. There is a fourth possible solution, which often appears in combination with one of the others. If the child is able to reach a clear understanding of the various difficulties, the sublimating process will then be more consciously and satisfactorily accomplished, and the emotions will be able to develop to their richest expression.

This transition stage is likely to be very difficult for the parents, who often have little knowledge of what is going on in their children's minds. Many parents make a dogged attempt to preserve the former relationship with their children, and so make it doubly difficult for them to find a new one. When children continue to feel and show the same affection and intimacy towards their parents, this behaviour will be considered as specially amiable and praiseworthy. But later on, at the time of an engagement or a marriage, all sorts of difficulties arise. The parents will be taken aback at finding that such a thing could happen in the case of their meek and yielding daughter, or of their excellent and affectionate son. It will probably seem to them extraordinary that other children, whose relations with their parents may have been more difficult and unpleasant, now seem to be able more easily to adapt their new emotional experiences to parental claims. Many parents are apt to drive out from their consciousness what they prefer not to see, for they find it an unpleasant experience, when the emotional changes during puberty begin to lead to the child's independence and detachment from home ties. Moreover if the natural development is hampered, we may meet with the Oedipus-complex in a more serious form than in cases of small children, because the conflict has been more completely driven back into the unconscious, and thus the strongly suppressed impulses will remain in a state of tension.

Even those parents who are aware of the necessity of this natural development, will find it a difficult task to help their children ; for while the child is longing for liberty to direct his emotions towards the outer world, he cannot entirely dispense with his old emotional centre, and needs love and care, although he can no more give the same undivided love in return. Great understanding and tact is required by the parents all through this psychic process ; and so this period of youthful life often runs a stormy course.

Another danger that belongs to the period of sexual maturity, is connected with the difficulty of choosing an object of the affections. At this age intimate friendships between young people of the same sex are very common. During this transition period the sexual tension is such that a physical touch may easily arouse sexual emotions, which may then be directed towards the same sex. Where intercourse with children of the same sex only is the rule at this age, such expressions of the sexual impulses cannot be wondered at. Homosexual emotions, sometimes psychic, sometimes combined with sexual acts, are a fairly common symptom, until a more definite form of expression can be evolved. Usually the attraction of the other sex will soon make itself felt, and then the emotions felt for the same sex will return to normal channels. But if these emotional relationships should continue for a long time, or if they are the result of quite early experiences in childhood, they may then lead to a fixation of the emotions, which may prove extremely difficult to re-adjust. Freud therefore considers neither this abnormality, nor the other perversities of the sexual life, as mere symptoms of degeneration, but looks upon them as disturbances in the normal development, usually brought about by circumstances (XI).

By way of recapitulation, I wish to draw the attention of those responsible for the education of children to the following three stages of development in the emotional life.

(1) In the first period contact with the outer world is as yet very slight, and it is of great importance to control the physical functions, suppressing what is useless and eliminating any wrong influences, because it will then be easier to prevent the emotions from finding a wrong channel of expression.

(2) The second period makes higher demands upon the educator, because it is now that emotional relations between the child and its surroundings are formed. Love has now become the most effective means of influencing the child, so it is imperative that parents should retain their children's affection and confidence. They ought to give an honest answer to any questions the child may ask, even about sexual matters; otherwise the child's confidence might easily be destroyed, and the influence of the parents would come to an end.

Experience teaches us that there is nothing to fear for those children, who have always received rational answers to their questions, and have thus been gradually initiated. If once their curiosity has been satisfied, they will not think so much about such matters as those children do who are left to search in the dark. The difficulty here is often on the side of the parents. Unless their attitude towards sexual questions is sufficiently natural and unprejudiced, they will not find it easy to enlighten their children in a tactful manner. Although love and confidence are most potent factors in education, parents ought to be on their guard against over-stimulating their children's love by sensual means. Too much tenderness, exaggerated caresses, frequent getting into bed with the parents, may all influence the child's emotions in a wrong direction by emphasising their sensual expression. Allowing a child to share its parents' bedroom too long may also have its dangers. No doubt any bad habit in the child, such as sexual auto-stimulation, must be discouraged. But what is most important during this period is that the child's emotions towards its environment should find new and better forms of expression.

(3) The third period coincides with puberty, when the parents are faced with the difficult task of helping the child to become independent and self-reliant. Satisfaction of the emotions must now be gradually transferred from the family circle to wider social relations.

We must not expect that these psychological discoveries of Freud will revolutionise education in the near future and shake it out of its usual routine. We can only hope to see great changes brought about when these new ideas have been more generally accepted. Our knowledge on this subject is constantly growing more exact as our data are amplified. Many details may have to be elaborated and revised ; but the chief points, as indicated in this chapter, will probably remain the same. I hope that notwithstanding this short and somewhat sûperficial treatment of the subject, I may have convinced my readers how important these theories are, and how useful it must be to gain a clear understanding of these intricate problems.

CHAPTER IV

THE ANALYTIC AND THE SYNTHETIC POINTS OF VIEW

BEFORE drawing attention to certain objections to Freud's psychology, I wish to recapitulate briefly the chief points of his theories.

According to Freud, all psychological phenomena, in their rich variety, are caused by instinctive impulses. The general trend of these impulses may be determined by heredity, but, within those limits, they are expressed in a great variety of ways. Those impulses which organise their forms of expression under the influence of the desires of the conscious self, may be said to constitute the conscious individuality, which is thus able to suppress the expression of other impulses that are inconsistent with it. These useless forces, whose expression has been suppressed, constitute the unconscious mental life ; and if they are few in number compared with those that constitute the conscious individuality, then they will probably cause no trouble, though they may give rise to some slight disturbances which find expression in dreams and in various character-traits. But if the suppressed element is important, it will manifest itself in morbid symptoms. The nature of these symptoms will depend upon all the various useless impulses whose expression was suppressed at a former stage. When an earlier form of expression has become " fixed," it will very likely be an important factor in causing morbid symptoms by means of regression.

It cannot be denied that these views on psychology often create an unpleasant impression. Freud was continually experiencing, at first much to his surprise, that the publication of his ideas had the effect of estranging the public and leaving him in isolation. Others have had the same experience. Discussions about Psycho-analysis, though arousing much interest, often produce an atmosphere of coldness and hostility. We must now try to discover why these theories create this unpleasant impression.

Freud's followers maintain that the resistance, which all of us feel to any exploration of our hidden impulses, must be the chief reason for our opposition to his views. I believe that this is true where the intensity of the hostile attitude clearly reveals its emotional basis. Some inner conflict is probably then touched on the raw by the theories of Psycho-analysis, as often becomes evident upon close investigation. So far, the explanation given by Freud and his followers appears to me to be right. All the same I consider certain objective criticisms to be reasonable. I can well understand that strong opposition has been aroused by Freud's terminology, by his wide use of the word sex, and by the careless manner in which his theories have been applied to insufficiently explored material. I have therefore avoided, as much as possible, the use of terms which might lead to misunderstanding: they are not essential to the new theories, and may well be altered and improved in the future. Such criticisms of Freud's work are justifiable, though they do not detract from the real value of his discoveries.

But there is a further important reason why many people oppose his theories. They cannot always define it clearly, and can only express their repugnance. This resistance would seem to be due to unconscious complexes: and yet this is not entirely the case The true reason is a difference of general outlook upon life. The character of Freud's theories clearly shows a pathological basis. It is true that he has also studied the unconscious life of normal persons as manifested in dreams and psychic disturbances; but this has formed only a small fraction of his material, and he has been apt to treat normal and pathological cases from the same point of view. There are many degrees of transition between the normal and the abnormal. Many abnormal conditions and traits are exaggerations of normal ones, magnified as by a microscope. In this way no doubt psycho-pathology throws a great deal of light upon normal psychology, and on various transitional stages between the healthy and the morbid. A neurologist does not usually meet with hostility when he confines himself to describing these transitional stages; but it is otherwise when he uses transitional symptoms as a means of judging normal persons, who are unpleasantly affected when they find such symptoms regarded as faults and frailties, in fact as signs of degeneracy. It is true that, if they are candid, they will admit these shortcomings; but they object to being judged and classified by means of them. They are right when they maintain that pathological psychology and normal psychology should be studied from different points of view. The function of a doctor, as of a policeman, is based on the assumption that there is something wrong in the world: his work only begins when some disturbance arises. Thus he is apt to judge everything from the point of view of the disturbance, or of the degeneracy of his patient, and his scientific training will urge him to trace these back to their origins. But the normal man approaches the problem from a different point of view. He is more concerned with what is right and successful than with what is wrong and a failure, and the idea of an ultimate goal is of more interest to him than a chain of causes and effects. The student of natural science only values the future in so far as he is able to find its causal connection with the past, and so to establish his causal laws. But scientific laws, and the past, only interest the normal practical man in so far as they help him to shape the future according to his desires; so he may well think that all this analysing and searching for the origins of weaknesses, is only of secondary importance, unless it shows how to build up a better future. Freud does not give us direct advice on this matter; he only throws light on the causal laws of morbid symptoms, and reveals the unconscious to the conscious mind, leaving his patients to find for themselves the guidance they require by looking into their inner mental life.

Freud realises that it is desirable to find new and more suitable fields of interest, to which the unconscious and repressed energies may be transferred. He calls this process of transference *sublimation.* But he leaves it to the patients to find their own way of sublimation, because he is convinced that any guidance by the doctor would be impossible without his obtruding his own views of life and his own manner of sublimation upon the patient. Freud confines himself to clearing away every obstacle to sublimation. Sometimes this method makes an unpleasant impression both on the public and on the patients, who are thus left to work out their own salvation. It is the process of sublimation which chiefly interests the normal person, and about which he desires to be enlightened. He does not ask, what is the cause of ill-health, but how he can keep healthy, or become healthy, and what are the best ways of development. Freud would say that the answers would be different in every individual case, and that everyone must find them for himself; otherwise he will become a copy of some general type and thereby lose his individual character. He would further expatiate on the difficulties inherent in the development of character, and so explain how certain traits and deficiencies are connected with earlier circumstances. To many people such theories seem discouraging, because they emphasise what is impossible rather than what is possible in human life.

Freud has given us a broader and deeper understanding of the human soul. Formerly its nature was conceived as being completely stable, and characterised by certain traits or attributes. Later on association-psychology taught us that all psychic events were caused by the interchange of atomistic-intellectualistic ideas. But Freud tends more and more to conceive the psychic life as the expression of various opposed forces which are continually being replenished from the unconscious background, and he has minutely described the development and inter-relations of these forces as they are manifested in the human emotions. Only in his last book (XVII, p. 34-41) has he treated the problem of the real meaning of life, and the forces that cause development. His answer is characteristic of his special point of view. He thinks that every instinctive impulse aims exclusively at reconstituting a former condition. Thus the desire for repetition would be the most fundamental power in living beings. The fact that changes have occurred in nature, is due exclusively, according to Freud, to external influences, and to the development of our earth and its relation to the sun. It is true he is objective enough to recognise that this view is purely speculative, and cannot be deduced from experience. He writes, "It is impossible to prove the existence of an evolutionary impulse in animals and plants, though it is also impossible to find arguments against supposing such a tendency." A little further on he adds, "But I do not *believe* in such an impulse, and I see no possibility of preserving this satisfying illusion." Whoever shares these views, will have to follow Freud to the logical conclusion he draws from them. If life has sprung from lifeless matter, and if all life's impulses are directed in the last resort towards reconstituting former conditions, then death, which is the return to the most primary condition, must be the real aim of life. If we agree with Freud in interpreting life merely as an adaptation to outward circumstances, we shall easily be convinced that the real significance of life lies in this last and most definite adaptation.

Freud considers that environment is the chief formative influence in the growth of the human mind. Thus, if the standards of civilised society did not early in life put a check upon the inherited impulses, they would create for themselves far wider fields of expression. It is true that he recognises that such checks and inhibitions as shame, repugnance or pity, may be in part inborn ; but to him they are just as much blind impulses as the other inherited instincts. It will depend on the child's milieu how far he will learn to harmonise these opposed forces. All the same, some of his inherited characteristics may modify this process. Thus a complicated temperament may cause special difficulties or unusual developments. The capacity for sublimation in each individual must largely depend on his physical and mental condition. All this is certainly one of the most practical and helpful of Freud's theories, for it is based on fact, and formulated accordingly, without wandering off into speculations which often prove misleading to students. Yet it seems to me somewhat onesided. I can best illustrate this by describing a similar problem in natural science. Darwin held that the complicated development of the various forms of life was due to environment, and to the struggle for life ; he tried to show the relation between every detail of the circumstances and of the corresponding development, and he rejected the idea that the development might be due to an inherent life-force which is always pushing on towards further expansion and evolution. Later scientists have proved the incompleteness of some of Darwin's theories, and further research has gradually convinced most men of science that, although the influence of environment must still be regarded as an important factor, it can no longer be considered as the only cause of evolution. Thus we are led to believe that life possesses some inherent force, which notwithstanding all the varying influences of surrounding circumstances, follows its own principle of development, and makes use of circumstances only in so far as they can be made to agree with this principle. This may explain the fact that an organ, such as the eye, arises in a similar manner in different animals, at different stages in their development, and under entirely different circumstances (II, p. 67). Bergson describes this life-force as a powerful vital impulse, the " élan vital," which is working throughout nature, and continually creating new forms in which to express itself.

The same problem of evolution can be found again in the microcosm of the soul. Here also new variations of form and expression are constantly arising, and though it is evident that past and present environment has a strong influence, yet it is doubtful whether these variations are in all circumstances exclusively due to environment.* I do not mean that a new variation might suddenly spring up independently of all surrounding influences, but that a guiding force may sometimes compel these various influences to work together in one direction. The question could be stated thus: does our desire for inner harmony belong intrinsically to the nature of the human soul, or is it caused by external influences alone? To put the question in a more psychological form: is the desire for sublimation a natural part of the human mind, or only the result of education? It is no doubt impossible to give an absolute answer to these questions. It depends upon our individual character, experience and general philosophy of life, whether we believe that all natural phenomena are subject to fixed laws, or that an inde-

* If one considers the inherited temperament as being a result of the influences of environment in former generations, we are again faced with the general problem of evolution.

pendent creative force may intervene. The relative value of these two beliefs cannot be measured by the intellect alone. Pure reason will never prove whether a mechanical determinist, or a creative indeterminist philosophy is the better (VII).

A believer in determinism holds that all the future is contained in the present, and will develop from the present according to fixed laws. In psychology this means that all psychic events have been completely predetermined by past and present circumstances which have influenced the soul. On the other hand, a believer in the free creative principle holds that, even if we could have full knowledge of all that the present contains, the future is largely uncertain and incalculable because, besides the mechanical laws, there exists in nature a creative principle of life, which, within limits prescribed by circumstances, is free to choose and create new forms. In psychology this would mean that in psychic events a human being *can* have a certain freedom of choice, and so may exercise a decisive influence on his mental development.

Scientists, in general, will feel inclined to hold the determinist theory, because they are occupied in finding causal laws for all natural phenomena, and therefore deny the possibility of freedom of choice. Even when investigating a process of evolution which never repeats itself, such as history, they are apt to apply their causal laws ; but they never completely succeed in explaining the process according to these laws. They express what Jung calls *nur das Nach-Wissen* (merely after-knowledge).

In opposition to the scientist's point of view, the practical man believes that within certain limits he is free to choose how he will direct his life. He recognises that his mental life is a process which never repeats itself in exactly the same way, and although ready to admit that he is bound by certain regular laws, he can never consider his free will to be a pure illusion. He feels within himself an independent impulse towards expansion, and if he is given to speculation, he will divine the presence of this spontaneous impulse in other forms of life. Several philosophers of our day (Bergson, Driesch, Vaihinger) do not accept the purely determinist point of view. The reader must turn to philosophical literature for a fuller treatment of this subject. I only wish to draw attention to these two divergent views of life.

The fact that Freud and his followers are apt to ignore this creative impulse, has caused a reaction in several psycho-analysts, who, both in their theory and in their practice, pay special attention to the sublimating process, and under the leadership of Jung and Maeder have founded the so-called "Zürich school of Psycho-analysis." This name is somewhat misleading, for the main point of their theory is synthesis rather than analysis. With them introspection does not merely serve to trace the origin and explain the meaning of mysterious desires and thoughts, but is used as a means to discover inner impulses of growth, which may be synthesised into a harmonious personality. It is true that this latter process is also recognised in Freud's psycho-analysis; but with him it is rather an indirect result of the treatment, and not the chief object. By attaining to a better understanding of themselves, his patients are naturally led to improve their mental organisation and to feel their way gradually towards better conditions.* The Zürich psychologists, on the other hand, concentrate upon this inner searching, and maintain that this can be done without endangering the objective nature of the treatment. Though they recognise the objections which have prevented Freud from working in this direction, they do not consider them insurmountable. They think that, although no general rules can be laid down as to how particular desires and emotions are to be sublimated, there are nevertheless various ways in which the human mind solves its difficulties, and that a clear understanding of these processes will help towards finding the best solution. The chief task of the synthetic method is therefore to explain to the patient the way in which, partly in his conscious and partly in his unconscious mind, this sublimating process is continually developing. It is evident that a satisfactory explanation of this kind can only be given after thorough introspection, as there would otherwise be a danger that the doctor might involuntarily impose his own opinions and theories on his patient. Intuitive guessing at the meaning of psychological phenomena would be as much out of place here, as when a doctor is trying to discover their origin in the patient's life-history. The way in which a dream is analysed, must depend upon the spontaneous association of ideas with the dream by the patient. In some cases these associated ideas will refer to the past, so that its connection with the dream will then be evident: in others they will refer to the

* Dr Ernest Jones, a follower of Freud, has written about the significance of the process of sublimation in education and in psycho-analytical treatment, but he has confined himself to indicating certain special points of view of general interest.

present in relation to various hopes and plans, upon which the dream may throw new and valuable light. In other cases again the association method may show that both past and present are referred to.

A few examples will illustrate the way in which the introspective material is made use of. Let us first take a simple case of forgetting. Someone has forgotten to post a letter, and now tries to discover the meaning of this forgetfulness. Suppose he remembers that the letter contains a promise of financial assistance to a relation, he will then realise that an unconscious avaricious motive prevented him from sending off the letter. Or it may have contained violent reproaches addressed to a friend, which on further consideration prove to be exaggerated or baseless, in which case the writer of the letter will be only too thankful that his unconscious feelings prevented him from sending it off. Thus in addition to many disturbing influences arising from the unconscious into the conscious, there are a number that are very valuable. Some people are easily susceptible to such influences, which may have an important effect upon their lives. We find this special influence of the unconscious mind not only in the inspiration of artists or scientific men of genius, but often in more ordinary lives. The publications of the Society of Psychical Research will provide any reader who is interested in this subject, with many striking examples. There he will find descriptions of dreams which revealed the place where a lost object could be found, or of cases when persons were warned of an approaching danger by premonitory feelings.

My next example will be a dream in which the

working out of an unsolved problem was continued. One evening a student had been reading a book about Einstein's Theory of Relativity, without completely understanding it. He had however grasped the idea that Newton's laws were upset by Einstein; so he made up his mind to study the elementary side of the problem more thoroughly. At night he dreamt that he went into a cellar where an Englishman, called Newton, whom he had once met on a journey, was occupied in soldering together two metal pipes, but was doing it in the wrong way. The dreamer felt anxious on Newton's account, lest his work should be criticised. As he turned to go away, he suddenly noticed various wires stretched from the pipes to the wall behind, and surrounding him in such a way that he had to cut them through before he could extricate himself. The shape of these wires was peculiar in being round at one end and square at the other.

When the dream was examined, the associated ideas soon made it clear that the acquaintance called Newton represented the great scientist, who, according to Einstein, had not done his work properly. The soldering of the pipes reminded him of a system of speaking tubes which he had seen somewhere, and which were going to be extended; this had seemed to him a stupid job, because he thought that a private telephone would have been a much more effective and up-to-date arrangement. Here we find the contrast between the old and the new system, just as with Newton and Einstein. The anxious sympathy he felt for Newton should be noticed, as it shows that the dreamer evidently felt more at ease with him than with Einstein. The necessity of breaking through the wires evidently arose from his having seen similar wires the day before in a workshop, where they served to connect some electrical apparatus (called " elements " in Dutch), and so might very well symbolise the elementary principles of Newton which imprisoned his mind. Thus the dream emphasised the necessity of breaking through this network before he could face the problem freely.

Here we see how an intellectual problem can be expressed by a dream, and how the search for its solution may be continued during sleep. In this case the dream did not really help to solve the problem ; yet this does sometimes happen, as I once experienced myself, when I was busy preparing a lecture but could not find a satisfactory way of treating my subject. After I had been puzzling over it, I dreamt that I was copying an etching, but that I felt I must emphasise more strongly the contrasts of light and shade. When I thought over this dream, it struck me that, a little while before, I had read a short abstract of the subject of my lecture, which at the time had seemed to me too flat and impersonal. The dream now revealed to me that I might use this article as a scheme for my lecture, only I should have to fill out and enrich the exposition.

It is such cases, which are concerned with intellectual problems, that reveal most clearly the creative and inspiring influence of the unconscious. But the unconscious may attempt to find a solution of emotional problems too, and it then often resembles a moral force working upon the human character. A curious instance of this is described by Peter Rosegger in his book called *Waldheimat* (IX, p. 317 and XXVII, p. 668).

"I usually sleep soundly; yet I have missed many a good night's rest, owing to my being haunted for many years during my simple life as a student and author, by the shadow of a tailor's life. It was not because I was always thinking about my past during the day; a thorough revolutionary like myself, who has cast aside his Philistine garb, can use his time more profitably. Probably I did not pay much attention to my dreams in my gay youthful years; it was only later in life, when I had acquired a habit of reflecting about everything, and when perhaps my Philistine side was re-awakening, that I began to notice that whenever I dreamt, I always imagined that I was a tailor's apprentice, and had been working for a long time in my employer's shop without receiving any wages. While I sat next to him busy with my sewing, I was conscious of not being in my proper surroundings, and I felt that I ought to be doing other things; but somehow an arrangement was always made by which I spent my holidays doing extra work for my employer. I often felt very uncomfortable about this, and regretted the waste of time. Besides I had to submit to scoldings and listen to reproaches, when my work was not satisfactorily finished. My wages were never mentioned. While sitting with bent back in that dark workshop, I often made up my mind to give up the job and go away. Once I actually gave notice, but my master paid no attention to it, and I went on working for him. How happy I used to feel when I waked after so many tedious hours! I used to make up my mind that if this persistent dream should recur, I would call out, 'It is only fancy. I am lying in bed, and I wish to sleep' And yet the next night I would again be sitting in the tailor's shop

"This went on with uncanny regularity for many years, until one night I dreamt that both my employer and myself were working at Alpelhofer's, the place where I had begun my apprenticeship, and that my employer was particularly dissatisfied with my work. He looked at me angrily and said, 'I wonder where your thoughts are wandering.' I thought that the moment had now come for me to get up and explain to him that I was only working for him out of kindness, and then to run away. But I could not do it. I did not resist when the employer took on another apprentice, and ordered me to make room for him on the bench. I moved into the corner and went on with my sewing. The same day another fellow was taken on. . . . There was no room for him to sit down; and when I looked up inquiringly at my employer, he said, 'You have no talent for tailoring. I dismiss you: you can go.' The shock of this remark was so great that I awoke.

"The morning light shone through the bright windows into my comfortable room. Treasures of art and luxury surrounded me on every side. . . . In the next room, I heard the cheerful voices of my children romping with their mother. It was delightful to rediscover this idyllic and peaceful life, so full of poetry and spiritual harmony; and yet I felt annoyed that I had allowed my employer to dismiss me, instead of giving him notice myself. The curious result was that from the night of my dismissal I enjoyed peace, and have never since been troubled by those apprenticeship-dreams about imaginary youthful years, which had cast such a dark shadow over my later life. My real youth had in fact been quite a cheerful and careless period."

These dreams of Rosegger presented a somewhat difficult problem to Freud. It was obvious that suppressed desires were not here seeking for gratification, for they were being gratified during the conscious life, and the dreams only recalled a life of humiliation and drudgery. Freud at first thought that their only significance lay in their relation to the past, and he compared them to his own dreams about working as a student in the chemical laboratory, which he used to regard as a particularly tedious occupation. For a long time he was in doubt whether to consider them as dreams of punishment for pride in a man who had been successful in life, or as the expression of a strong desire to be young again. He was at first inclined to hold the latter view (IX, p. 320), which however was strongly attacked by Maeder (XXXVII), who pointed out that it is difficult to find a satisfactory explanation of the feeling of relief which Rosegger always experienced when waking up, if his early life had been so attractive. Nor is it easy to understand the liberating effect of the last dream, unless we assume that Rosegger's fame and worldly success had tended to make him feel proud and vain. These weaknesses, though threatening to poison his mind, created at the same time a reaction in the depths of his delicate poetical soul, which resulted in a continuous striving to conquer such evil tendencies. This was expressed by the sense of humiliation felt by him in his dreams. The dismissal, and the consequent feeling of liberation, would mean that he had conquered his snobbish pride and vanity. If we consider the dream from this aspect, we shall find that it symbolises a fragment of the poet's moral development, like other similar dreams that symbolise the soul's strivings after inner harmony.

After rejecting this theory for a long time, Freud has lately declared his acceptance of it, but with one reservation: he does not believe that such dreams originate from repressed unconscious backgrounds of the mind, but from what he calls the "preconscious" mind.* We must however be careful not to confuse such processes with those other preconscious processes which can easily be transferred into the conscious mind. With many people this kind of psychic process never becomes conscious.† We owe a debt of gratitude to Jung and Maeder for drawing attention to this matter. The right understanding of these unconscious processes is most important both from a theoretical and a practical point of view, although Freud and his followers do not attach much importance to this side of psychology. Here again they have been influenced by their attitude towards pathological

* Freud's paper on "Erganzungen zur Traumlehre" at the Sixth International Psycho-Analytical Congress at the Hague, September 1920.

† I am glad to find that Tansley (XXXIII, p. 53-56) has also noted that Freud's distinction between the preconscious and unconscious is in this case unsatisfactory. Tansley considers the unconscious does not consist merely of repressed unconscious processes, but is chiefly composed of what he calls, the primary unconscious. According to him, "the primary unconscious is to be regarded as the basis of the entire mind, as the centre or core of the psychic organism. The mental elements corresponding with the great primitive instincts are originally seated in this region, and from it the psychic-energy which activates the complexes of the foreconscious is continually welling up."

psychology. They aim first of all at eliminating morbid symptoms in their patients by discovering their origin through the historical-analytical method; and so the history of such symptoms is more important to them than the meaning. When the patient's symptoms reveal some intention, this is often merely the intention to be ill, and so escape from some difficult problem—the so-called "escape into illness." No doubt such intentions may not give us much information about the nature of the illness itself; all the same we are not therefore justified in considering all expressions of the unconscious merely from this point of view.

Every process in a living organism can be looked at either from the historical and causal side, which will reveal its connection with the past, or from the actual side, which will throw light upon its future development. When we explain a machine or a scientific theory, we describe how it is used and for what purpose, and we may leave out the historical origins as of little importance to our explanation. But if we wish to explain the meaning of the Nelson Monument, or of the coronation of a king, the historical side will necessarily be emphasised, while the use made of them will be unimportant. Freud and his followers, being chiefly interested in the historical side, are in danger of misunderstanding those psychic processes in which the other side is the more important. During the actual treatment of patients this danger may be small; but even then it is important to discover what are the real aims of the patient, and what their possible value may be as a factor in his particular phase of development. But the narrowness of Freud's theory is most apparent when the historical-analytical method is applied to the normal and healthy mind, which is constructive and synthetic in character. Symbols in art and religion should in Freud's view be reduced to nothing but expressions of suppressed emotions, chiefly of a sexual nature. We admit that further enquiry into the history of the human mind may prove that the sexual impulse has been a great factor in the development of religion and art ; and there are many facts that point that way. All the same it cannot be maintained that mere analysis and reduction will lead us to a full understanding either of art or religion. We may be thoroughly acquainted with the history of religious symbols or of art, and yet be very different from the religious man or the artist, who daily use these symbols as the formative elements of their lives. There is a constructive force in human intercourse, in art and in religion. They educate man towards clearer and more beautiful forms of self-expression. In order to make use of these forms, it is more necessary to gain an insight into their meaning than to understand their historical origins. Even if we assume that the sexual instinct has contributed towards developing these symbols, the wonder is that the sexual impulse, instead of retaining its most primitive form, has gradually developed such very different modes of expression. Interesting as the history of this development may be, it will teach us less about the real nature of these symbols, than the actual experience of them in our present life can do.

The dreams of Rosegger suggested to us that the constructive interpretation of dream-symbols might be of great importance. We saw that lately Freud has been inclined to accept this point of view, though hesitatingly and with reservations. On the whole he seems to consider these constructive dreams to be very exceptional. Not long before he wrote very decidedly (XV, p. 61): "A dream does not want to tell anyone anything: it is no vehicle of communication; on the contrary, it is constructed so as not to be understood. For this reason we must not be surprised or misled, if we find that a number of the ambiguities and vagaries of a dream do not permit of determination." Thus Freud regards dreams merely as a kind of safety-valve for suppressed tension, of which the immediate and undisguised expression could not be accepted by the conscious personality. Jung and Maeder on the other hand consider that in both normal and abnormal cases the constructive analysis of dream-symbols is of great value, as it reveals the dreamer's endeavour to solve his difficulties, and that this ought never to be overlooked. All the same, while a mere historical interpretation will often lead to erroneous conclusions, we must be on our guard against seeking for a constructive meaning in every dream. Maeder distinguishes between dreams which act as an outlet for suppressed tension, and those which search after some solution (XXVII, p. 673), but holds that the condition of the soul is symbolised in all. Works of art may also symbolise both the relaxation of tension and the search for new forms of expression.

This double meaning of symbolism has been clearly explained by the Viennese psycho-analyst Silberer (XXXI, p. 665). He points out that a symbol can only be regarded as such, if we try to discover a further meaning behind it, which is usually more complicated than the symbolic image. Before we can say that a mental image A is really a symbol of the thoughts B, C and D, the mental image A must have been further analysed and differentiated.* Now there are two occasions when A may be regarded as A and nothing more. First, when the more detailed interpretation leading to B, C and D might be painful or unpleasant. In this case the symbol A has been selected for reasons of sentiment. This happens in repression. Secondly, when someone is too unintelligent to express a complicated mental concept, his want of intelligence will then make him choose the symbol A, which in his case is the only form of expression suited to his stage of development. The human mind is only capable of grasping a certain proportion of truth at each stage of its development, and will resist any higher demands. Thus we find in the old alchemy-lore an intricate mixture of chemical and psychological knowledge, that later on became differentiated into chemical and

* Silberer says that a symbol A may be used to express an idea B. This may lead to misunderstanding, for it seems to me that a symbol is always trying to express something of a complex nature. Ernest Jones in his article on "The Theory of Symbolism" (XXII, p. 129) indicates that a symbol is chiefly a substitutive representation of a definite unconscious image. This view seems to me to result from his somewhat narrow theory, which only attaches value to the historical side of a symbol. By using this arbitrary restriction, the solution of the problem given by Jones is deceptive. Though he agrees with Silberer that symbols may occasionally be a factor in a sublimating process, he is chiefly interested in those symbols which do not succeed in this process, but appear as substitutes for the sublimation aimed at. In my opinion he does not sufficiently emphasise the important rôle of symbolism in the history of humanity as a bridge between old and new forms of expression. He expresses his disbelief in all creative evolution (p. 173), and therefore concludes that the explanation of symbolism as expressing a development or striving towards new forms, is wholly unscientific (p. 179).

psychological-philosophic theories, which diverged ever further and further, until each acquired a complete terminology of its own (XXXII). Another instance is the idea of re-birth, which, when we look into it closely, is found to be a symbol of intricate psychic processes. We often cling to old symbols, because of historical tradition, or because our sentiments are thus gratified, or owing to a suspicion that there may be more in those symbols than has yet been explained. Thus the alchemist parables may possibly contain some spiritual lore, which the new psychology has not yet unravelled.

If we admit that the mind is in a state of modified, or rather diminished consciousness while dreaming, it seems reasonable to suppose that, apart from any repression, the same thoughts, which appeared in a clearly defined form by day, may appear as symbols in dreams. These symbols will arise because the dreamer lacks control over his thoughts during sleep. I may here remind the reader of the dream about Einstein's theory which I referred to above.

Freud has admitted that the choice of symbols by the unconscious may be due to its peculiar way of expressing itself, and not merely to repression. Yet it seems to me that his attitude towards symbolism is influenced by his theory that the choice of symbols is determined by sexual repression, otherwise he would surely have been able to find a greater variety of meanings in fairy tales, myths and popular sayings. For instance, the symbol of sacrifice is common throughout the world, and expresses the necessity of giving something up in order to attain to something higher. The profoundest interpretation of this general law of life is not found in the domain of sex, but is clearly manifested in religious symbols. Throughout history we meet with symbols of a general nature, which, far from having a merely sexual significance, have continually assisted the human mind in its search for new forms of expression. Symbols are the chief means by which the human mind expresses, not so much those ideas which it has outgrown, or wishes to conceal, but those which it has not yet mastered.

Thus every symbol has a twofold aspect. It may express a regression, a backward movement, which leads us away from a clear conception. This happens either under the influence of a strong affect, such as occurs in neurotic repression, or else in a state of diminished consciousness, such as is produced by fatigue or sleep. Both cases present a condition of collapse and diminished potentiality. We find the same phenomenon in social psychology. During periods of collapse the human mind falls back upon symbols, which are apt to be made concrete and so lead to dogmatism and convention. But new ideas also tend to clothe themselves in symbolism. Every idea and every synthetic emotion which is not yet clearly defined, needs a symbol for its preliminary expression. Instances of such symbols are the communist state, the superman, the "élan vital." Here the symbol will be a sign of progress, as when at the call of some watchword, a man throws himself into some vague project, which may be of a religious, social, artistic, or mystical nature. The influence of such symbols is specially felt at a certain period of youth; and we find their clearest expression in the ecstasy of poetry and religion. Nietzsche expressed this in striking words: " My brethren, take note of the hour when your spirit wants to speak in parables; that will be the beginning of your virtue." Such symbolism is a sign of exaltation and ardent vitality.

We now have two keys for the interpretation of symbolism: historical reduction or *causality*, and the discovery of the intention or *finality*. If we take the view that the symbol is only in appearance an attempt to express something definite, but is really nothing but the outlet of uncontrolled impulses, and is therefore merely " something primitive," the danger will be that by thus reducing the symbolic material to its simplest form, we may overlook its more interesting side. On the other hand, if we try to discover in the symbol some mystical, elusive meaning which cannot be more clearly defined, and which we feel bound to treat with the respect we owe to all hidden sources of life, we may make the dangerous mistake of attaching some deep and valuable meaning to symbolic material, the importance of which is merely historical, and so fail to realise that this meaning is not inherent in the symbol, but is put into it by ourselves.

Both these dangers are met with in the interpretation of dream-symbols. The followers of Jung and Freud are as usual the extremists in this matter. Some followers of Freud hold that all symbols are a disguised expression of repressed sexual tendencies. It must be admitted that Freud himself is partly responsible for this opinion, as he has always concentrated the whole of his attention upon the analytical side of both dream-symbols and general symbols, and is chiefly interested in tracing their origins from primitive instincts.

He admits that there is room for the other point of view, but considers that it is superficial, that it will fail to teach the patient anything new, and may often give rise to fancies which will hinder him from finding a genuine solution of his difficulties. Freud may well be right about this in the actual treatment of many cases; but he is not justified in his general condemnation of the synthetic method of interpretation, and it is quite possible that the adoption of his view may lead to serious misunderstanding of the dreams of some patients.

Jung and Maeder on the other hand consider that both dreams and general symbolism may reveal new ideas and new aspects, though expressed only in vague symbolic form. They agree with Freud that it is impossible to interpret the whole of dream-symbolism by means of the association-method, and so they regard the dream as a primitive form of expression of the human mind. But they adopt a wider point of view than Freud, when they relate the significance of these symbols to the history of civilisation. Thus they sometimes discover a similarity between the problems that occur in the development both of individuals and of the human race (XXIV, XXVIII, XXXII). There is some danger that this method of interpretation also may be applied too narrowly, for every psychical phenomenon has a history, but not everything that has a history is necessarily capable of development. Enthusiasts of this school may be too ready to find a profound meaning in every dream-symbol, and the analysis of dreams might thus easily degenerate into washy mysticism or superficial moralising, and lay itself open to ridicule and contempt.

It will need great circumspection to avoid these dangers in actual practice. Our standpoint, when we are interpreting a dream, ought to depend both upon the associated material provided by the dreamer, and upon his general condition. When we are treating such complicated material as the human mind, it is always dangerous to work according to a set scheme. A dream, like every other psychic product, is connected with the rest of the mind by innumerable threads, and these connections can never be satisfactorily expressed in a simple formula. This complication also makes it difficult to give satisfactory illustrations of dream-symbolism, for the interpretation of a patient's dream is only a small fragment of the psycho-analyst's vast field of observation. It is almost impossible to select and define any part of the intricate and coherent structure of ideas and images which are provided by the patient in connection with the dream, without destroying the greater part of this cohesion. When we relate an analysis of a dream, we are like a traveller, who wishes to describe to his friends a country which is completely unknown to them. However exact his descriptions may be, he will never succeed in giving a perfectly clear picture.

All the same I will try to give illustrations of these two standpoints of interpretation. My first instance is the dream of a patient who at the time seemed much inclined to give up my treatment, and to seek a cure in work for which she was making somewhat extravagant plans. She was also much exhausted by anxieties and difficulties. One night she dreamt that she was lying in a cavern under a hill, in which she was imprisoned, and from which she could find no way of escape. She felt too weak to search, and had the feeling that she had been lying there for a long time. She felt her strength was slowly ebbing away, and thought that she would probably die of exhaustion. Then she suddenly noticed an opening in the roof of the cavern, through which someone, whom she recognised to be myself, was looking at her. She thought that the opening would be too small to let me through, but though constantly overcome by a feeling of faintness and exhaustion, she noticed that I was succeeding in reaching her. She could not exactly tell how, but I managed to draw her through the narrow opening, and when she looked around, she found herself in my house, lying on a bed, naked. I was searching in a cupboard to find her some clothes, but could not find anything that would fit her. She felt somewhat stronger and thought that she had better not stay any longer; but as no clothes could be found, she had to go out naked.

In my opinion the real value of this dream cannot be discovered by the association-method, and no associated ideas were given me by the patient in this case. In order to avoid undue elaboration, I will interpret these images without attempting to justify each interpretation. We can take this dream to symbolise the idea of birth. The dark cavern which contains the weak and helpless dreamer, the small opening through which she emerges with difficulty, and the curious fact of her being naked at that moment, will then all become clear. According to Freud, the dream would be the regression to a childish fantasy, which probably had its origin when the child was discontented with its lot and imagined itself returned to the mother's womb in order to be re-born under more favourable circumstances. For the dreamer, these circumstances would be connected with her treatment in the doctor's house to which she comes after re-birth.

It is doubtful whether this interpretation takes into account all the important aspects of the dream. In the first place it does not explain why the dreamer should have the dream at this exact moment; nor are the other points, such as the impossibility of finding clothes and the necessity of returning home, made much clearer. It may help us if we compare this birth-fantasy with similar symbols in history. The idea of birth as symbolising a re-birth, and as indicating an inner spiritual change, has played an important part in the religious creeds of nations of very different kinds. My patient was undergoing a similar spiritual change at the time of her dream, and this would explain the reason of its occurrence just then. If we consider the dream in this way, we are struck by the fact that her unconscious attitude towards the treatment is very different from her conscious attitude. In the dream she is excluded from the influences of the outer world, from which she is consciously expecting a solution; and the doctor's influence, which she consciously resists, is all the same of assistance to her in her difficult re-birth. A possible explanation of her being unable to make use of the doctor's clothes, might be that these new clothes symbolise a new relationship to the outer world, so that the dream would express her feeling that she cannot simply adopt this new relationship directly from the doctor, as then it would not fit her particular needs.*

The other dream which I have chosen, also contains some symbolic images that cannot be interpreted by the association of thoughts and recollections, although the dream was related to an occurrence of the previous evening. The dreamer is a musician who suffers from the fact that he loses the mastery of his instrument when playing alone in public. Consequently he has never attained as much success as his talents would lead one to expect. He is well-read and intelligent, but has led a somewhat solitary life owing to various circumstances during his youth. He seldom expresses his feelings, but when he does so he is usually very vehement. He has always been inclined to take a sceptical view about ideals, and professes to admire science alone. After a discussion on religion in which he took a strongly anti-religious line, I lent him two books on Hindu philosophy. These interested him very much, and he read them till late in the evening. That night he dreamt that he came into my consulting room, and told me that a sentence in one of the books had seemed to him entirely unintelligible. It ran as follows: "When the murderer believes that he has killed a man, or when the murdered man believes that he has been killed, both ignore the fact that the soul cannot murder or be murdered." Then he dreamt that I laughed and said I would try to explain it to him. The room then changed; everything remained in its place but became transparent like crystal. He was able to look far away through the

* I must add that I had never talked with the patient about re-birth or any similar subjects.

walls, and seemed to be surrounded by space. It was very beautiful and impressive. He looked around, but could not find me, and then he realised that I also had become transparent. He now saw that he would not be able to reach me, and awoke with a mixed feeling of anxiety and admiration.

The patient could only add that he had really read that sentence in the book, and had found it difficult to understand. The obvious interpretation is that the dreamer's unconscious mind was working at the difficult sentence, and that his dream symbolised this search for an explanation, which he felt to be beyond his grasp. It is also clear that the sentence was specially difficult to him, because it assumed the possibility of an independent spiritual existence, an idea entirely alien to his sceptical materialistic attitude. His attempt to approach this conception was symbolised in the dream by the way in which the material world became transparent, for spirit is popularly conceived as transparent matter. It was natural that he should think of this in my consulting room, because he wanted to question me about it, and also because it was the place where he had gained some understanding of his own spiritual independence. In this way we can regard the dream as a continuation of a rational process in a psychic domain, where thoughts are more naturally clothed in images.

But some points in the dream remain untouched by this explanation. It is not clear why the dreamer hit upon that particular sentence about murder, as there were many other references to the spiritual life in the book. Nor is it clear why I should disappear, and why he should feel anxious. We should have expected that he would discover me in these new spiritual surroundings, and that this would have given him satisfaction. It is a curious fact that these points are related to two dreams which he dreamt a short time before. We know by experience that successive dreams are sometimes connected, if the mind, in between, has not been influenced by some disturbing event. So I will point out the connection between this dream and the two earlier ones, though it would lead me too far to give a full account of them. In the earlier dreams also someone had laughed, but in both cases this had so infuriated the dreamer that he had killed the person who laughed. Here we find the problem of murder which is the starting-point of the third dream. The later part of my treatment had revealed that the patient was more dominated by these passionate feelings of hatred and rage than he would admit, and that they probably had a strong effect on his relation with his audience, when he appeared in public. The mere idea that anyone should laugh at him was enough to arouse these passionate feelings. After the dream had been interpreted, several memories arose which showed what an important part these feelings had played in his early youth. In the dream the laughter is not followed by murder as before, but by matter becoming transparent and by my disappearance. We know that Freud considers disappearing to be the symbol of death; and if we accept his view, it is clear that in the last dream the images of laughter followed by disappearance or death have the same murderous significance as in the former dreams; but this was not expressed, because here it would clash with too many of the patient's feelings, and so was only expressed by the sentence about the possibility of murder. His anxiety about my disappearance would thus mean his reaction against his passionate feelings of hatred. This interpretation may seem somewhat far-fetched, but we must remember that a man who has an exaggerated fear of being laughed at or despised, has usually a strong sense of his own importance. While he is giving a truthful and detailed account of his life, he may easily imagine that the doctor is laughing at him, and may feel hurt and resentful. Other feelings towards the doctor may repress his resentment; but it may all the same find expression in his dreams, though usually in a disguised form.

By these illustrations I have attempted to show that there are two entirely different methods of interpreting dreams. How can we decide which is the right one? They seem to represent two entirely different points of view, two opposed outlooks on life. The answer should be that both are right, but that neither of them can contain the whole truth, and that they cannot be brought into harmony with each other, because each points in a different direction. It is like two men on a road, one always looking forward, the other backward. Each sees a different landscape, and their description of the road will be true in either case, yet entirely different. The attitude of each patient towards his own problems must determine whether we should interpret his symbolism chiefly from a prospective or from a retrospective point of view. Any ideas associated with the dream-symbols will also naturally influence our interpretation, and this association-method will often reveal a tendency in the dreamer to compensate for the narrowness of his conscious views of life. But the psycho-analyst who relies entirely on the purely scientific point of view, and is only concerned with the retrospective side of dream-symbolism, is in great danger of misinterpreting the meaning of a dream in which prospective symbolism predominates.

In my last instance the dream was the first sign that the relations between the patient and his fellow-men were undergoing a radical change. The feelings of hatred, the fear of being laughed at or of being badly treated, are expressed, as well as the attempt to find more satisfactory relations. It is remarkable that this change of attitude during treatment is often specially noticeable in the patient's relations with his doctor. He is the object on whom the patient can practise his feelings. Thus the real significance of the dream is that it does not so much reveal the prospective or retrospective point of view in the dreamer's mind, as the inner change within him, which is an attempt to harmonise these two aspects. The old wild feelings of resentment tried to force an outlet for themselves, just as they did in the earlier dreams. But something now intervened. The meaning of the sentence in the book was, " You cannot kill: that is an illusion." But why? It was I, who in his dream, showed him the reason; and it was here in my room that his outlook on the world was widened. It was both crystallised and grew more spiritual, and consequently the motives of his resentment and hatred towards me gradually disappeared. This illustrates the way in which the two sides of dream-symbolism can be brought into harmony, and only by means of such a harmony can we find an interpretation of dreams of this kind, which does full justice to their content.

Freud in all his investigations applies his causal-historical theory, so he naturally emphasises the past influences which unconsciously govern the present psychic event. The actual form in which these influences are expressed interests him less than their origin, and their expression appears to him merely as a camouflage of unconscious desires. Jung, on the other hand, lays special stress on the importance of this expression of desires. This appears to Freud and his followers as a return to the old theory, according to which dreams and morbid symptoms are the simple automatic expressions of actual psychic processes. But they do not perceive that Jung is able to incorporate Freud's historical method into his own interpretation, while his attention remains chiefly directed towards the dreamer's actual conflict and its solution.

I must repeat that it is a mistake to try to discover such deep meanings in all dreams. Many dreams, if not most, are simply outlets of various kinds of tensions, which are caused by repressed emotions. But when these special dreams occur, which symbolise the solution of the dreamer's difficulties, a true and clear understanding of their meaning will considerably advance the solution of many other psychic problems, which their misinterpretation will tend to retard.

Later on I hope to consider how far the theory of the unconscious, and of its relation to the conscious mind, is affected by our recognition of this impulse towards sublimation, and by knowledge of the various ways which lead to it. Here I only wish to trace the influence of these new conceptions upon psycho-analytical treatment. We have seen that psychic products such as fantasies and dreams sometimes possess a constructive meaning, which indicates a possibility of psychological development. They thus show some resemblance to the inspiration of artists and inventors, which reveals a creative function in the unconscious mind. This wider outlook brings new light, but also a new danger. The theory may be exaggerated in practice, and so lead to endless arbitrary interpretations. The great advantages of psycho-analytical methods can only be realised, when the doctor takes a purely objective attitude and abstains from any form of suggestion. This is difficult enough when he is tracing back the psychic content of dreams to its origins; but it is much more so when he tries to discover in his patients the constructive and sublimating impulses, which constitute their process of growth. The temptation to use suggestion is always strongest in connection with one's ideals and views on psychological development. Suggestion and direct teaching may of course often be useful; but they must not be confused with strictly psycho-analytical methods of investigation, which are meant to be helpful by an objective statement of the truth. To deal properly with synthetic psychology, we must first be thoroughly acquainted with analytic psychology and the construction of the mind. Even then there is a danger that we may be tempted to lose our objective point of view and wander away into the morass of dilettantism and quackery. What is needed is that the new synthetic psychology should be based upon a sufficiently scientific and comprehensive theory of psychic development. The next chapter contains some account of the results of the latest medico-psychological experiences.

CHAPTER V

PSYCHOLOGICAL TYPES

NEW methods of education are now being explored in all countries. The old system has not been entirely abandoned, but its weakness is so evident that even those who still cling to the old school, recognise that a thorough reform is needed. Many principles, which used to be regarded as infallible, are now being given up. In old days the child's mind was considered to be plastic like wax, so that it could provide a suitable material upon which the educator could exercise his talents. Nowadays we pay more attention to the rights of the child's nature. We try to discover his own particular line of development, and to eliminate any disturbing influences, such as social pressure, which might interfere with his freedom of growth. But we must not confuse such freedom with aristocratic individualism. The ideal of freedom, whether in education or in social life, often comes into conflict with the ideal of equality that forces the individual to surrender his own rights in favour of the rights of the community. Freedom for one often means lack of freedom for another, and so causes inequality; while equality necessitates some sort of constraint. A just compromise between both principles is the only solution, but it is rarely met with. The educational ideal which emerges from this conflict, attempts to satisfy both the need for freedom and the need for equality. Its realisation will mean that all children would have equal opportunities of development ; but at the same time education will have to adapt itself so much to the individual needs of the children, that no special or exceptional line of development need be suppressed. Even should economic conditions allow such ideals to be put into practice, there would still be the question whether the demands made upon the teacher would not prove to be too great. He will not only need a thorough knowledge of all the various claims of society, so that he can gradually prepare the children to adapt themselves to their life in the community, but he will also need a delicate understanding of the children's various temperaments and the difficulties connected with each. He will need special tact besides, if he is to apply his knowledge in the best way, so that the children may develop along independent lines without undue pressure from the teacher. Only thus can the combined ideal of general and individual education be realised. The educator will have to shape the child's surroundings in such a way that the child may find in them what he requires in each stage of his development. Thus the educator will have to become himself a part of these surroundings, rather than the sculptor who desires to model the child according to a design of his own. Freedom is the means, not the aim. The aim must always be development, which implies the idea that the child should learn to adapt himself to the lack of freedom that exists in the world. It is therefore of the utmost importance that the educator should thoroughly understand and sympathise with the inner life of his pupil, so that he may have a clear vision of the child's tendencies and struggles. Only under such conditions will the teacher be able to develop the child's conscience and self-confidence, while allowing his special talents to attain their full growth.

Although there are many practical difficulties in the way, it is probable that an increasing number of people will devote their best powers to the service of such ideals. Perhaps the most serious difficulty is due to the differences between human beings, and the narrowness of human character. It is surely due to differences of temperament, that people so often misunderstand and torture each other with the very best intentions and principles. If all these disagreeable mistakes could be avoided, the world would become a much pleasanter place to live in. This not only applies to adults, but more particularly to children, who often become the victims of unsuitable education. The knowledge of these mistakes and injustices sometimes induces educators to throw all principles overboard; but this will not improve matters, and will only lead to chaos. The real solution would be that instead of formulating the principles of education in easy ignorance, we should remodel them with a view to special forms of character. For this purpose there is great need nowadays of a true understanding of types of character and of their individual needs. Anyone seeking enlightenment on this subject from official psychology, is likely to be bitterly disappointed. Hitherto psychology has been chiefly concerned with the investigation of the intellectual and perceptive processes of the mind, with the object of laying down as many generally valid laws as possible, in imitation of natural science and its exact laws, where great results have been obtained by starting with simple processes which can be repeatedly observed and tested. Now the intellectual and perceptive processes, because they are less directly influenced by the whole personality, are more easily isolated for the purpose of investigation than the emotional processes, which are more complicated and differ more from one another. The result has been that comparatively little attention has been paid to the emotional life, which is nevertheless of the greatest importance for the study of character types. Freud, though he has added so much to the psychology of the emotions, has concerned himself very little with the problem of classifying character types, but, led by his practical experience, has been chiefly interested in the origin of various mental disturbances. His medical point of view has emphasised problems and difficulties rather than their possible solution, and so his psychology is of little use for a classification of character. All the same human character is constituted by such solutions and sublimations far more than by its failures and difficulties. It is true that suppressed tendencies and emotions may give a certain colour to the character ; yet it would be an exaggeration to say that the whole character is dependent upon them. We have seen how Jung and Maeder, in their treatment, draw special attention to sublimations and their origins and inter-relations, and how Freud has objected to this on account of the danger of suggestion. This objection may be valid and useful in practical treatment; but in theory such one-sidedness cannot be justified.

However great may be the importance of recognising the individual type, and allowing it to develop in its own characteristic way, no one can deny the possibility of establishing the general validity of certain definite principles of psychological development, and of certain practical rules for dealing with it. The whole science of education is based upon this possibility. Otherwise all educative influences would have to be imposed upon children from without, regardless of the way their minds are constituted. To take another instance, an important side of religion aims at assisting our inner strivings; and if these strivings were utterly different in each individual case, the influence of religion, which only aims at a general solution, would then merely have a spoiling and distorting effect. Freud and his followers are apt to make a bugbear of "the schoolmaster" and "the parson." This fear is not wholly unwarranted, and is shared by many other people. Both pedagogy and religion have too often relied upon dogmatic claims, and thus have done violence to the growth of the mind. All constructive psychologists must be on their guard against a similar error. The Zürich psychologists who are consciously aiming at a synthetic psychology, are aware of this danger, which they try to avoid by closely examining the actual and potential characteristics of each individual, in order to collect sufficient material to build a general theory as to the aims and possibilities of development. In this they clearly differ from the theologians and pedagogues. But of course the individual solutions at which they aim have a close relation to the more general solutions; and thus the two schools of thought influence each other, in a way which may prove of great benefit to psychology, pedagogy and religion alike.

PSYCHOLOGICAL TYPES

In defence of his synthetic psychology Jung has pointed to other sciences, such as synthetic chemistry, which tries to construct new combinations of matter, in contrast to analytical chemistry, which aims at reducing composite matter by the shortest possible method to its component elements, and deduces the qualities of composite matter from its elements, and from the laws according to which its elements are combined. Synthetic chemistry, on the other hand, though it too is based on these elements and these general laws, aims at applying and combining them in new ways, so that attention is specially directed to the difference between the various ways of forming new composite matter, and to its new specific qualities. To continue the comparison, a synthetic chemistry that is not founded on the laws of analytical chemistry would be an impossibility Anyone who tried to work at synthetic chemistry without a thorough knowledge of analytical laws, would resemble the muddle-headed alchemists of the middle-ages. Psychological synthesis without analytical knowledge would be equally dangerous. The comparison fails in one point: the psychological process is not so much a construction as a growth; and intuition may make it possible for us to enter imaginatively into this process of growth without thoroughly understanding it, whereas such intuitive methods would be utterly impossible with any chemical process. All the same, if psychology is to help us to a truly scientific understanding of our needs, it must be based on analytical knowledge, and not merely on intuition. A synthetic psychology can only be formulated atter analysis has furnished us with extensive knowledge of spiritual development.

K

The most important part of Jung's work is his classification of certain psychological types. In contrast with Freud's typical forms of failure, he is more concerned with typical ways of sublimation. We must begin by distinguishing between the original disposition of a human being, and his special character, which is the product of his development. A character is always a complex whole : it appears as an organised entity, which is not yet revealed in the original disposition. The organisation and unity of the developed mind is not merely the result of the repression of what does not fit in with the whole ; for when we compare its psychic content with that of a child or savage, we find that the difference does not consist merely in the repressed parts. The conscious development of an individual is the process of differentiating his original forms of expression when he is forced to find new adaptations. This process will bring into harmony various contrasts which at first appeared irreconcilable. For instance, when a child or a savage insists on realising all his desires, there will be an impassable gulf between his selfishness and the general interest. This selfishness may become circumscribed and differentiated by the force of circumstances. He may come to insist upon some only of his thoughts, feelings and purposes. In so far as he does this, some of his own interests will then be merged in the interests of the community, and this will lead to a solution of the conflict. To take another instance : a man may have a very quarrelsome nature, and at the same time feel a great need of affectionate relations with other people. These two sides of his nature will constantly give rise to inner struggles and conflict with his surroundings, until he has found a wider and more general interest, for which he can work in union with others. A similar synthetic development may be observed when someone is endeavouring to find a more stable outlet for his sexual needs.

In the course of his investigations Jung was struck by the fact that the individual adaptation, which leads to differentiation, varies greatly in different people. He was thus led to distinguish two groups, which he named the *introvert* and *extravert* types. Introverts are those persons who have an inwardly directed mind, and whose life is governed by their inner needs. We must not however identify this with selfishness, for the inner nature is not merely selfish ; it often calls for sacrifices, and it desires love and friendship, forces which impel men to live for others. People of the introvert type are not exclusively governed by their own needs, because they are forced to take the circumstances of their environment into account. But when different possibilities of action present themselves, they will choose rather to be led by their own feelings and opinions. Of the two worlds, the outer and the inner, with which the psychic life is concerned, it is the inner world which will be of most importance to the introvert. The laws of the inner world may be seen most clearly in certain psychic processes, such as fantasy or a logical train of thought, although they may contain some factors borrowed from the outer world.

Persons of the extravert type are primarily concerned with adapting themselves to their surroundings. They cannot of course entirely ignore their own disposition, but they specially develop that part of it which is considered useful and desirable by the surrounding world, without taking into account the satisfaction of the most important needs of their own nature. Their attitude of mind is turned chiefly towards the outer world, and their psychic life is governed more by their sense-perceptions, than by inner needs and laws.

Both modes of adaptation are indispensable to every living being. A person who only takes into account his own instinctive needs, without adapting himself to the claims of the outer world, would be incapable of satisfying those very needs, and would die of starvation. On the other hand, one who completely adapts himself to his surroundings, without making any attempt at selection, would submerge his own individuality and waste all his energy in being tactful.

In the unconscious or partially conscious condition of the animal mind, the balance between these two adaptations is naturally maintained; for nature takes into account the necessity of both. In man, this balance is often upset by the conscious mental life. If once our attention has been drawn to this distinction, we shall easily notice the more pronounced instances of either type. It will be found that most people belong rather more to one type than to the other, governing their life either with a view to their surroundings or to their inner needs.

After Jung's practical experience as a neurologist had led him to distinguish between these two mental attitudes, his attention was drawn to another important factor, the predominant mental *function*, which together with the predominant mental *attitude* are the two chief influences that determine the form of adaptation. Further investigation led Jung to distinguish four primary functions, which he could not differentiate any further. These functions, which co-exist in the mind of every individual, *Thinking*, *Feeling*, *Intuition* and *Sensation*, have long been recognised and distinguished by psychologists; but Jung was the first to point out that their effect will vary enormously according to whether one or another is predominant. For instance, if a person is chiefly guided by his feelings when trying to adapt himself to daily life, his thoughts and sensations, and also his actions, will be strongly influenced by his feelings. This would apply also to the predominance of any other function.

In order to understand the relations between the functions, we must first consider the psychic life of primitive man, and conceive the content of his mind as centred round the unconscious instincts which are the supreme governing force of his psychic life Consciousness at this stage appears rather as a by-product than as a dynamic factor. There is as yet no will, no conscious striving, no sense of responsibility. The fragmentary psychic events are governed by Sensation and Intuition, in the form of impressions and impulses. The unity and logic of the conscious civilised man is still lacking; and the primitive mind allows many conflicting elements to exist in it side by side, which would not be possible at a later stage of development. Besides the instincts, the primitive mind contains some vague knowledge about the object of its instinctive activity, and it will also be vaguely aware of its subjective attitude towards this object. These elementary functions however will be still mingled in an indistinguishable whole, nor will they always be found in equal proportions. If at any moment some obstacle prevents or delays the instinctive activity, then the thinking and feeling functions will get an opportunity for being developed; activity will then be turned either into Thinking or Feeling. Thus we see that the primitive mind, though mainly governed by chance impulses, also contains some rudimentary forms of Thinking and Feeling. This leads us to consider the relations of these functions to Sensation and Intuition. It is a mistake to regard these latter as the immediate symptoms of instinctive life. Between the instincts, as we find them manifested in animal life, and Sensation and Intuition, lies the borderland of the unconscious psychic life. This borderland of unconscious processes is a development of the original instincts, which conditions Sensation and Intuition. Sensation does not mean a merely passive receptivity to all impressions; it also contains an unconscious choice, which is determined by the general character of the individual. In Intuition, the influence of the unconscious is still more clearly seen; intuitive action or perception is still more obviously determined by the unconscious process of discovering a certain meaning or connection behind a given fact, and of moulding and adapting this fact to personal needs. The unconscious processes of choosing, discovering and combining in Sensation and Intuition, lead to an immediate experience of conviction; but it is seldom possible to discover the grounds on which this conviction is based. If we try to penetrate into these unconscious origins by a difficult and elaborate introspection, we may meet with some curious psychic processes which are very different indeed from conscious rational processes. This has led Jung to adopt the term *irrational* or empirical functions for Sensation and Intuition, as contrasted with Thinking and Feeling which he calls the *rational* functions.

Both Thinking and Feeling are functions concerned with sorting and organising the conscious material of the mind. Their activity presupposes the existence of Sensation and Intuition, which provide the material of the psychic event; but this material is systematised and classified by Thinking and Feeling, each using its own method and its own standard of values. Hence the name rational, which is given them by Jung. He writes (XXXIV, p. 659): " *Rational* means the reasonable, or that which corresponds to reason. By reason I understand an attitude of mind, the essence of which is to shape thought, feeling and action according to objective values. These objective values are established by the average experience of facts both of the outer world and of the inner life. . . . The rational attitude which enables us to recognise the validity of these objective values, is not the product of a single individual's mind, but of the whole history of mankind. Most objective values, and also reason itself, are firmly welded complexes of conceptions which have come down to us from remote ages, and have gradually been organised through countless thousands of years with the same inevitableness with which a living organism reacts to the average constantly recurring conditions of its environment, confronting them with the corresponding function-complexes, such as the eye which completely corresponds with the nature of light. . . . Reason therefore is the expression of man's adaptation to the average event, and this adaptation has been gradually developed into closely-organised complexes of conceptions, which determine the objective values."

Thought and Feeling differ greatly in their ways of organising the conscious material. Thought is concerned with sorting and classifying sensations and impulses, so as to form a general survey of both the inner and the outer world. It finds it necessary for this purpose to restrain spontaneous and immediate reactions, and replace them by the psychic process of systematising actions and sensations. Feeling, on the other hand, organises both sensations and impulses under the influence of some psychic attitude, while at the same time this psychic attitude is expressed and worked out through the organising process. Whereas Thought aims at defining and sorting its material, and then organising it into one objective system, Feeling combines and develops its material into a synthesis. Thought consists of surveying various possibilities of action, while Feeling leads to one complex action, which unites in itself these various possibilities. If an unpleasant remark is addressed to a thinking type, he will usually, before he answers, consider various possible ways of reacting. He may either reply with a retort, or he may point out the rudeness of the remark, or else he may try, by turning the other cheek, to persuade the other that he was in the wrong. In a similar case the feeling type may react by combining all the above possibilities into one expression.*

* Readers of Jung's book may notice that my views upon certain theoretical matters are somewhat different from his. According to Jung, the function of Feeling is essentially one of valuation. This definition seems to me insufficient, since other functions are equally capable of assigning values, which may be either accepted or rejected by the individual.

These various forms of psychic activity seem to be always competing with one another; they are never equally powerful in the same mind. Each of these functions is capable of independent growth and development, that is to say they are able to loosen the bonds which originally held them together and become differentiated. Other functions will be suppressed only in so far as they interfere with the leading functions. I will now describe the nature of these differentiated functions.

Sensation is the psychic function that draws the perceptions into the conscious mind, both those which we obtain from the outer world through our senses, and those which arise from our inner physical condition or its changes. Sensation is an element in the mental image, since it supplies it with the perception of its object. Sensation is also an element in Feeling, because the quality of Feeling is largely determined by the bodily and mental condition. In its original form Sensation is always mixed up with images, feelings and thoughts, and may then be spoken of as concrete Sensation. It may also become differentiated as pure and abstract Sensation, in which case it will control the other psychic functions and suppress those that might interfere with it. It may also control the conscious will, which may then be said to become subject to an æsthetic mental attitude. To the artist especially this abstract Sensation is of great importance; and susceptibility to such impressions and emotions is one of the most precious possessions of the human mind. In those cases where Sensation is overshadowed by Intuition, Feeling, or Thought, sensations will very often fail to reach the consciousness; while those with whom Sensation is predominant, will assimilate into consciousness as many impressions and emotions as possible.

There is a great difference between extravert and introvert Sensation. In the extravert type, Sensation is dominated chiefly by impressions received through the senses, while in the introvert type, it is the inner sensations caused by these impressions that are predominant. We must be very careful not to confuse these inner sensations with feelings They are not the feelings themselves, but an original element in them. The feelings are a product of conscious activity, as we shall see later on, when we treat this question more fully.

To persons who are primarily of an extravert sensation type, the sensuous impressions of the outer world are of predominant importance. It is what can be seen, heard or touched that is of value to them, and influences their actions. They are easily susceptible to pleasure and grief, and they have great power of æsthetic discrimination. On the other hand they are very dependent on their surroundings, and so their activity is chiefly reactive.

If Sensation is introvert, the mind is chiefly influenced by the inner sensations. An instance of this type is the artist who approaches his work exclusively from the subjective point of view. The more our sensations are differentiated, the more clearly shall we be able to appreciate what has eternal value for humanity. Man possesses a certain inherited need of Sensation, and the more he gives his sensations free play, the better will he be able to distinguish those which respond to his inmost nature. In these cases of passive receptivity, all that happens is that the inner sensations are differentiated and clarified but not further developed. This inner mental activity usually remains hidden from the outer world, and only those impressions which touch the inmost being, can bring about a reaction. The value of this function in its developed form, may be said to consist in a sensitiveness to what has eternal significance, arising from the profound needs of human nature. When this type of mind is very pronounced, its onesidedness will become evident; such persons are too passive, too much aloof from the world, and find a special difficulty in self-expression. In consequence they often give the impression of not having found a satisfactory way of sublimation or adaptation.

Intuition is the spontaneous active expression of the instincts, and of that part of the unconscious psychic life which is most closely related to them.* Intuition may mean a certain manner of perceiving or formulating ideas; but it may also manifest itself in feeling or action. Intuition itself is not actually either Thought or Feeling, but it is, as it were, a primitive psychic function, which contains elements of Thought and Feeling. It presents a complete psychic content, the origin of which cannot be derived from other conscious contents. It brings with it its own immediate conviction of certainty. In their primitive forms, Intuition and Sensation are difficult to distinguish. The distinction is one between spontaneous impulse as opposed to susceptibility to impressions. But

* The name is derived from *intueri*, to contemplate. As names for new ideas are generally chosen by men of intellect, it is not surprising that the intellectual side of the function is emphasised in the word Intuition.

impulse is always stimulated by impressions, while susceptibility is nearly always combined with a tendency to react to these impressions in a certain manner. When Intuition is differentiated, it becomes more abstract. The psychic life will then grow to be further removed from Sensation, while Feeling and Thought will be only permitted so long as they do not disturb spontaneous expression. The mind then consciously attaches great value to spontaneous insight and inspiration, and aims at being led by sudden impulses, which it is always ready to accept. On the other hand susceptibility to impressions is much diminished.

If Intuition is combined with an extravert attitude, then the individual will form intuitive judgments of what goes on in the outer world, and will be apt suddenly to discover connections between things, without being able to explain them. Such judgments, and the actions and expressions of feeling resulting from them, are sometimes surprisingly justified later on by events, or by a roundabout process of reasoning. While Sensation is chiefly concerned with the actuality of things, Intuition sees what is of personal importance. It is specially gifted in discovering all the various possibilities of individual development and activity. Even in cases where Intuition is not the leading function, it is often capable of finding a solution where no other function could succeed. Jung writes (XXXIV, p. 527): "If Intuition predominates, all the ordinary circumstances of life seem to be enclosures, out of which Intuition must find a way. It is always seeking for new paths and new developments of life in an outward direction. All circumstances soon appear to the intuitive mind as a prison, or as an oppression, which causes a longing for liberation. Things in the outer world seem at times to acquire an exaggerated value, when they can be made use of for the purpose of a solution, or a liberation, or the discovery of new possibilities. But as soon as they have served as a bridge or ladder, they seem to have lost all value, and are cast aside as unnecessary lumber. A fact is only valued in so far as it may contain new potentialities, which may outgrow the original fact and serve in turn to liberate the individual. Possibilities, that arise suddenly, become compelling motives to the intuitive mind, and it will sacrifice for them everything else." In contrast with the advantages of this rich variety of possible activities, we find the disadvantages of such qualities as changeableness, fickleness and lack of harmony.

While extravert Intuition deals with possibilities of the outer world, introvert Intuition sums up psychic events in images, which have a subjective value and significance, and express inner possibilities. These images appear as spontaneously as the judgments of extravert Intuition, so that sometimes the images and convictions are not recognised as having their origin in the individual's own mind. This applies not only to the hallucinations of the insane, but also to the inspiration of artists, prophets and saints. Nietzsche, for example, is said to have felt as if his Zarathustra had been dictated to him by someone else. But as men's minds are nowadays chiefly directed towards the outer world. we usually meet only with inferior expressions of this function. The value of such inspirations is more likely to be appreciated by artists or by persons with deep religious feelings. The fact that our instinctive disposition is made up out of the deposit of the experience of innumerable preceding generations, makes it seem possible that such products of Intuition are of great value. If the intuitive function predominates, inspiration will be looked upon as the most valuable psychic process. Sometimes this inward contemplation is looked upon as an aim in itself; but it can only be called a form of sublimation if the object of contemplation has some general or personal significance, which will probably be of an artistic, moral or religious kind. The disadvantage of this intuitive function is the vagueness which it frequently shows. Its predominance in the individual will often lead to muddle-headed mysticism and over-confidence in the subjective point of view.

We have described *Feeling* as the development of a psychic attitude or reaction. This can be applied to both the sensational and the intuitive side of Feeling. Both in Sensation and Intuition there is a relation between subject and object, which can be described as an attitude of the individual towards his perceptions. This attitude may be shortlived, variable and superficial; or else it may be durable, unvarying and intense. It is only in the latter case that real Feeling arises. All prolonged or intense sensations and intuitions are accompanied by Feeling, although it need not necessarily be conscious or clearly marked. If the feeling is a durable one, or if it is very intense, the contents of the personality are more and more drawn into its sphere and assist its development. In intense sensations and intuitions we see this effect as emotion. The influence is then felt throughout the body and mind; the heart-beat is accelerated, breathing becomes irregular, the colour comes and goes, and the limbs sometimes relax or contract spasmodically. Even memory, thought, judgment and will, in fact the whole imaginative life, may thus be influenced. If Intuition and Sensation are spread over a long period, the result will be a mood This kind of Feeling can be described as a grouping together and a becoming conscious of all the various processes of which it is composed. Thus Feeling in its primitive form is never unalloyed. Only where Feeling is the leading function, will it become differentiated and pure, and will then gradually dominate the whole psychic life. The individual will feel an imperative need to have a stock of these developed feelings ready to meet all emergencies, and he will attach an absolute value to these feelings. He will tend to link up his experiences into a harmonious and synthetic whole, which will be strongly coloured by Feeling. He will value and assimilate everything that is consistent with his feelings, and reject everything else. These feelings, as they become independent of Sensation, Intuition and Thought, will tend to dominate the whole psychic life, and will be spun out to an infinite variety, which may be expressed with great subtlety and plasticity.

In the extravert type, Feeling depends chiefly upon the outer world, and the individual will feel a wide range of contact between himself and his surroundings. His life will be influenced, not so much by overpowering emotions and moods, which are the expressions of non-differentiated Feeling, but by the desire to bring his perceptions, thoughts and actions into satisfactory relation with the outer world. He will readily express his feelings, and so endeavour to create a harmonious atmosphere of which he stands in urgent need. His expression of feeling will arouse similar feelings and moods in others, and he will often show great skill in this process of suggestion. His own complexity and delicacy of feeling will enable him to understand the feelings of others, even when they are imperfectly expressed. This understanding may not always be conscious, but it will appear in his reactions; and all these various qualities will help him to get into touch more easily with others. The danger will be, that in order to obtain a pleasant relationship, he may unduly suppress other valuable sensations and intuitions, and sometimes allow the objective truth to be obscured, so that his Feeling comes to be satisfied with the mere semblance of things.

The introvert feeling type is more interested in his inner harmony. His deep emotions and moods are often hidden from the outer world, except in the case of an artist, who may reveal himself in delicately sensitive expressions and actions. The feeling introvert, like the sensation introvert, is inclined to shield himself from the influences of the outer world, and allows only what satisfies his inner needs to act upon his mind But his sensations and moods will be much more highly organised and developed, than would be the case if Sensation alone predominated. His inner life will be more individual and coherent. His attitude towards the problems of life will determine which sensations and impulses he will accept or reject. The rich complexity of his feelings will enable him to find certain ways of sublimation, but he will adapt himself almost exclusively to his inner life. This adaptation is of no immediate social use, unless he expresses himself in art or in religion. The unhappy fate of being misunderstood is often the result of this lack of outward expression.

Thinking aims at rejecting the personal influence, and tries to formulate an objective system in which it can classify the products of Sensation and Intuition. Both Sensation and Intuition contain an element of knowing, as well as an element of Feeling. This element of knowing is abstracted by Thought, when Thinking becomes the leading function: otherwise it remains more or less mixed up with the other functions. Our knowledge is made comprehensible by being grouped into a system of ideas. While Feeling rejects or accepts according to its psychic attitude, Thought does so in accordance with the facts which it has recognised and systematised. Undeveloped Thought is Thought that is still intimately mixed up with Sensation and Intuition. Only gradually does Thought become differentiated by rejecting what does not belong to pure Thinking. It does not merely deal with facts, but also aims at classifying impulses and feelings according to their general usefulness, or in obedience to an intuitive appreciation of their comparative values. It is always endeavouring to formulate a system of objective impersonal values. Ethics too is one of its main products.

Although both extravert and introvert Thinking are thus concerned with fixing values, we find that their different attitudes will produce very different results. The thinking extravert classifies his sensations, according to the opinions and ideas of the outer world, and of his social surroundings. He also systematises by Thought the life of the impulses, valuating it according to principles borrowed from his surroundings. He tends to neglect the claims of his inner disposition for the sake of his experiences of the outer world. Material facts are what chiefly govern his mind, and when his Thought groups these facts into an objective system, the result will often be a materialistic view of life. As this system is obviously not the direct product of his own inner needs, it will usually not be a very living one, but of a somewhat formal nature. A man of this type unconsciously makes the mistake of transferring the immediacy of his external sensations to his method of dealing with his experiences. If his extravert attitude is strongly marked, he will tend to neglect more and more the assimilation and development of experience, so that the final result will be a confused and overwhelming mass of disconnected facts. We find striking instances of this in the present state of many sciences. It is natural that the thinking extravert should be in danger of becoming dogmatic, when he attempts to group his impulses according to popularly accepted standards of value. When he is treating facts alone, he may attain very valuable results; but when dealing with sensations and impulses, he has to assimilate the opinions and principles of many different people, in order to attain a sufficiently wide point of view of his own. Thought alone can be of little help to him here, for he must rely on principles borrowed from his surroundings, and thus the only valuable result is the systematising of these principles.

The thinking introvert will deal chiefly with the actualities of his inner nature, and try to fix laws and principles for his actions. All the same he can deal with external sensations, just as the extravert thinker can deal with mental experience obtained by introspection. But just as in such a case the thinking extravert confines his interest in the main to outward symptoms and to what he hears from others, so the thinking introvert will be more influenced by subjective feelings and convictions when he is dealing with external sensations. He will accept the objective truth of his perceptions only in so far as they agree with his theories and with his system of grouping his perceptions. Accordingly his method of dealing with external experience has less objective value than the method of the thinking extravert. On the other hand it has two advantages. Firstly the introvert's system of grouping experiences will be more alive and creative, because more light is thrown on the subjective element by a deeper analysis, and the thinking introvert always feels himself at home in abstractions Secondly, for the purpose of establishing objective values, the introvert will derive more help from his own introspection than the extravert, who tends to rely on outward symptoms and the information of others. All the same there is a danger that the introvert may over-estimate the general validity of his own specially systematised experience, and so may form wrong judgments about the experiences of others, and fail to take advantage of their corrective influence.

When dealing with intuitions, which appear in the form of impulses and feelings, the thinking introvert will aim at a kind of subjective economy rather than at discovering universally valid principles. He is more conscious of the subjective nature of his judgments than a thinking extravert, and will admit almost too readily that his judgments have only an individual value. He bases them upon self-knowledge, carefully measuring and balancing every impulse and feeling. This over-cautious method may sometimes destroy his activity and spontaneity. Thus there is a danger both of his becoming sterile, and too obstinate and theoretic in his opinions, because he spends too much thought upon the search for a right line of conduct.

Before I describe the psychological types resulting from the predominance of the differentiated functions, I must draw attention to their inter-relations. In the first place we must remember that there is no clear line of demarcation between the several types. These functions are all present in every human being, and it is often more difficult to distinguish them in imperfectly developed persons, or children, although even then a distinct superiority of one function or of another is often to be found. We must also remember that when one function predominates, all the other functions are not suppressed to the same degree, because they do not all present such a contrast to each other as Thought does to Feeling, or as Sensation does to Intuition. It usually happens that there is a secondary, less developed compensating function, which helps the personality to adapt itself in a different direction, so that when the predominant function is extravert, the secondary function is introvert, and vice versa. But as the secondary function is always the weaker, the chief function is often made use of, even where it is out of place. Certain functions are more useful for some adaptations than for others. For instance, Thought is particularly effective at testing various facts and possibilities by means of experience, so that theoretical and practical science is the special domain of Thought. Feeling is useful in order to establish harmonious relations in the outer and the inner world. Extravert Feeling, which develops both sympathy with others, and the expression of personal feeling, is of great value in all human relations, and also in the interpretative arts. Introvert Feeling, on the other hand, enables men to enjoy the rich variety of their inner nature. Intuition plays an important part, when mere experience is of no help toward establishing sympathetic relations with others. It is the function that discovers new ground, as for instance in creative art, or in commercial affairs. Sensation is of great importance to the artist, and we owe to it the power of enjoyment in general.

It sometimes happens, as I have said above, that the success of the leading function tempts us to use it for purposes for which it is less appropriate. When this proves a failure, we either have recourse to some less developed function, or else imitate other people's expression of the appropriate function, which usually means that we adopt a conventional behaviour.

A man of the thinking type, whose wife wishes to go to a party, to which he does not want to go himself, will first try to persuade her by reasoned arguments that it is better for her not to go. He may next use various conventional expressions of feeling to support his case ; and finally he may lose his temper in order to convince her. This all happens because he has been unable satisfactorily to express his feeling that he wants her to stay with him, in such a way that he can influence her feelings.

A lady of the feeling type falls ill. She refuses to send for the doctor, which would have been the obvious thing to do, but persuades her husband to stay at home and neglect his duties. She then dismisses a servant because she has been so unfeeling as to break one of the best plates. The next thing that happens is that she sends for some medicine which had done so much good to the mother of a friend in an illness that was rather like her own. Finally, she will perhaps go to a quack, in order that he may cure her by the old method of laying on of hands. Such behaviour is mistaken, because nothing that she chose to do could have led to any useful result. Feeling was first called upon to effect an adaptation, and when that proved inadequate, recourse was had to primitive or conventional behaviour.

Sensation and Intuition, being less complicated functions, are not in such marked contrast with each other. Neither of them conveys to the mind the elaborately developed conviction which is given us by Thought and Feeling. If either Sensation or Intuition be the leading function, it may happen that a slavish subjection to the other less developed function will serve as compensation. For instance, a merchant, who shows extraordinary intuition in conducting his business, and understanding the characters of his colleagues and assistants, will sometimes become the blind slave of a beautiful woman who is entirely unsuited to him. He may also throw up some important plan, merely because he feels out of sorts for the moment; and both in his business affairs and in his sexual life, he may be scrupulously bound by convention, while completely neglecting it in other matters. In this case subjection to certain elementary sensations and to conventional ideas acts as a compensation. Another instance is the man of artistic feeling, who wishes to enjoy life in peace, and yet may suddenly give way to an impulse, which will force all sorts of unpleasant duties upon him. He will feel bound to observe some religious or social discipline which will interfere with his enjoyment of life; or he may suddenly disturb the pleasant atmosphere around him by some unexpected impulsive outburst. His excessive receptivity will thus be disturbed by some conventional idea, or else by an intuitive impulse.

The predominance of one function at the expense of the others, may not only hamper development by giving rise to primitive or conventional forms of expression, but it may also be the cause of more serious symptoms such as neurosis. Jung has shown that such neurosis often arises when the tension of the predominant function becomes too great, because it is being used in a case where some other fully developed function could alone have brought about a satisfactory solution, whereas now this secondary function in an undeveloped form is forced to express itself unconsciously, thus disturbing the conscious mental activity. This view is so far in agreement with that of Freud, who also recognises this onesided type of development, though his work is more concerned with the problem of what factors and processes have interfered with the expression of the unsublimated feelings and desires. Jung, on the other hand, is more interested in the compensating activity of this undeveloped part of the personality, and tries to trace its attempts at development. He considers that not only such manifestations of the unconscious as dreams and psychic disturbances, but also certain morbid symptoms, are all expressions of a desire to get rid of a conscious onesidedness. He quotes Nietzsche to prove that nervous symptoms can be of great use to a man, because they may force him into some kind of life, where he will find fuller opportunities for developing what is valuable in him, and will not be tempted to waste his powers in unproductive by-ways of activity. Jung writes (XXV, p. 296) : " There are people the meaning of whose life—whose real significance—lies in the unconscious ; in consciousness lies only all that is vain and delusive. With others the reverse is the case, and for them the neurosis has another significance. An extended reduction * is appropriate to the one, but emphatically unsuited to the other." For people of this kind, Jung advises a synthetic treatment, which aims at bringing the meaning of such unconscious processes into consciousness and so developing their possibilities, rather than an analytical treatment, which checks these processes by tracing them back to the originating desires and circumstances. I shall deal with the relation between these conscious and unconscious processes in a later chapter.

I will now describe in somewhat greater detail the characteristics of the various types, and will begin with their most pronounced forms.

* *i.e.* of the morbid symptoms.

A person of the *extravert feeling* type is dominated by feelings, which are aroused by the outer world. Probably this type is most pronounced among women. The centre of their psychic life lies in their emotional relations with other persons. They realise imaginatively their circumstances and feelings, and are able to put themselves completely into their place. It was this type in fact, which Jung originally regarded as the real extravert type. They feel that their emotions possess an objective value, and they find support for this feeling in the fact that others are affected by similar emotions, and that the world generally ascribes certain values to them. They experience an overwhelming need to test their emotions by those of others, and to find agreement if possible. They are very unhappy when they are out of touch with their surroundings, and show great ingenuity in finding new ways of getting into touch with them. If they cannot find sympathy, they prefer strife to mere indifference. They are specially adapted to life in a community, and feel at home in any form of society where they can find personal contacts and maintain elaborate emotional relations. Though a difficult situation may sometimes make them feel awkward, yet they do not suffer from shyness, for they are too sure of being able to adapt their emotions to circumstances. Since more varied opportunities for such adaptations are offered by intercourse with human beings than by lifeless nature or animals, they will avoid solitude and prefer such enjoyments and sports as can be shared with others.

The feeling extravert has a special gift for expressing the most varied shades of emotion, so that others may be able to share his feelings. Accordingly we find that the most famous preachers and orators, and the most talented actors belong to this type. When our attention is drawn to a woman of this type, it is not so much by the emphasis with which she expresses her feelings, as by the delicacy with which the expression is adapted to the occasion. She will never say or do anything that might disturb a harmonious atmosphere; on the contrary she will help to create and maintain it in all sorts of little ways. Feeling extraverts can never remain mere spectators when anything happens which touches their feelings, but will take part in creating the emotional environment by their active sympathy. Thus the French, who have developed the expression of feeling to such a high degree, translate the verb "to be present" at a ceremony by "assister" (XXIX, p. 141). Persons of this type also show their desire to share in the lives of others by continually making engagements and seeking new acquaintances.

They have moreover a gift for expressing their thoughts as well as their feelings, and so they often show a decided talent for teaching. Some writers have maintained that all thinking is done in words; and though I do not believe this to be always true, yet it seems to be so in the case of the extravert feeling type. They think in a dramatic form, as if they were addressing an audience. Their thoughts and emotions do not come into existence until they are expressed, but arise through and during the process of expression, which consequently often seems lengthy and clumsy to a rapid abstract thinker. Their thoughts well up and flow onwards while they are addressing their hearers, a faculty which is of great advantage to orators and lecturers, since it makes their speech more living. But it is difficult for them to be brief and businesslike in their communications. The fact that Thinking is dominated by Feeling tends to blur their thoughts, although they may often be expressed in beautiful images and rich oratory, which will appeal to the heart and imagination of the audience. The thoughts of persons of this type will not carry so much conviction as their feelings. Although they suppress Thought when it comes into conflict with Feeling, yet they cannot be said to be unreasonable people. They often show much practical intelligence, because they can vividly realise other persons and circumstances, and know what they are aiming at themselves.

Their activities also are much influenced by Feeling. Their outward appearance will often reveal the nature of the feelings that dominate them, as may be seen in a well-bred lady or a clergyman, as well as in demi-mondaines and degenerate aristocrats of this type. Their actions become more and more influenced by their predominant feelings, which they have a growing desire that other people should share. They wish to prove to everyone that their feelings are the right ones, all the more if there is some doubt as to whether general opinion is on their side. When driven by powerful feeling, they are able to exercise a great influence on their environment, especially if they meet with sympathy and support among those around them. But usually their feelings are not so much expressed in striking actions, as in the creation of a harmonious emotional atmosphere.

They see themselves and their own lives only as they are reflected in their relations with others, and in the opinions of others about themselves; and so they are very sensitive to praise and criticism. Encouragement will greatly strengthen and develop their emotional reactions, while contradiction, or criticism that is difficult to answer, often has a most depressing effect upon them. Owing to their extravert tendency, they possess no inner certainty and conviction. Superficially they often give the impression of only caring for outward appearances. But we must remember that they have no other means of knowing or of changing themselves, than by observing the attitude of their neighbours and trying to harmonise their own desires with their environment. Thus it is through an outward harmony that they will find the way to an inner harmony. But there is a danger that they may cleverly manage to bring about this outward harmony, without really changing themselves as much as ought to be necessary for the purpose. It is quite possible for a feeling extravert to be an extreme socialist or communist, and yet at the same time to be living in idleness and luxury.

While the characteristics of this type may be of great value in practical life, this is sometimes counterbalanced in pronounced cases by certain disadvantages. For instance they find it difficult to form businesslike judgments, a failing which is usually considered to be characteristic of the female sex. The personal side of their emotions is very important, all the more that they are not conscious of their subjective attitude, but are convinced that their judgment is objective and of general value. As this personal side is unconscious it may lead to all kinds of conflicts which are quite incomprehensible to them, and make them look for the cause in other people instead of in their own character. Another set of difficulties is caused by the various feelings becoming markedly differentiated, so that they may feel drawn in various directions. They are always living on their outer selves, on their points of contact with other people; and they fail to concentrate on their inner selves, where they might compare and readjust their divergent feelings. Morbid symptoms may arise, especially where the conflict between acts and feelings is in strong contrast with the desire for harmony. Here they will unconsciously try to satisfy this desire for harmony by ignoring their spiritual needs; and the thoughts, sensations and feelings, which were suppressed in order to preserve harmony, will find a disguised outlet in morbid symptoms. Hysterical patients, such as those described in the first chapter, belong mostly to this type. I agree with Freud that these expressions of the unconscious contain everything that was thrust away as useless from childhood upwards. But we should also admit Jung's view that the impulse of the unconscious towards expression and consciousness indicates an incipient desire for compensation. This means that the feeling function, which tried to repress everything for the sake of harmony, is thwarted so as to make room, though very imperfectly, for some other function. Inner harmony may be found by Thought; and Jung interprets some of the dreams of hysterical patients, and their desire for solitude, as an incipient attempt to find a solution by means of a hitherto unused function. In order to find such a compensating function, a systematic introspection, which aims at making everything conscious, will be of the greatest use.

Persons of the *introvert feeling* type find support and direction in life by developing the subjective side of their feelings. This type also is chiefly found among women. They resemble the other introvert types by the fact that their outward appearance and conduct reveal very little of their inner life, so that introvert types are much more difficult to distinguish than extravert. The way in which they resist outside influences is often more characteristic than their positive expressions. The mask behind which they hide, is a simple, gentle attitude, childlike or sometimes melancholy, which may give the impression of coldness or indifference. Superficially, one would never consider these people to belong to the feeling type; for when moved by feeling they become quiet and absorbed, and if ever they express themselves, they do so only after they have worked out their emotion within themselves. Thus they are very often misunderstood by their neighbours. They carefully hide their emotional life from others, and only express it by secret piety, or else in poetry, which they are very unwilling that anyone should see Usually they feel a secret desire that some day the rightness and excellence of their own feelings should be acknowledged by others. In some cases they tend unduly to assert their own feelings by indirect means, not so much by communicating and suggesting them to others, as by obstinately resisting anything that might interfere with them. They may be justified in this resistance, because it is founded on a delicate emotional motive; but their manner of expressing it is not adapted to the outside world, and for this reason proves unsatisfactory.

In the lives of such persons we constantly meet with this inconsistency between motives and their expression. Thus when they express their feeling in a poem, they will weigh their words very carefully; on the other hand they will often neglect the ordinary forms of politeness, which have no meaning for them, or else they will hide behind some simple conventional form of expression. Sometimes indeed their delicate feelings will appear, and create an impression of intimate contact, which however may be suddenly broken off.

The feeling introvert is not affected by the opinions of others about himself; he judges and values his feelings according to a subjective standard of intuitive convictions. The warmth and confidence, which the extravert feeling type can impart to everyone around him, remains enclosed in the inner mind of the introvert, providing him with a refuge in case of difficult or unpleasant experiences. Such persons seldom give the impression of great activity; for circumstances will not often offer them the right opportunity for actualising their inwardly elaborated feelings, and they hardly ever succeed in creating circumstances for themselves They accept the fact that they must remain misunderstood.

They do not see the world as it really is. The feeling extravert adopts only a certain part of the outer world, and disregards all the rest: but the attention of the feeling introvert is concentrated on whatever comes into contact with his inner emotional needs; and as he is acutely conscious of this conflict, he seldom ventures to show his feelings, which he imagines no one could ever appreciate. A feeling extravert, when he is lacking in adaptation in any direction, is never conscious of it; whereas a feeling introvert will be very much aware of the fact that his own feelings often do not correspond with their expression. Yet although he takes a sufficiently critical view of himself and others, the result will not be a better adaptation, but rather the undermining of his self-confidence. He will assume that others are as critical as himself, and he may grow to regard the outer world as malignantly hostile; while the consciousness that his life is passing by joylessly, may lead to fear and melancholy. Both in this case and in the case of the thinking introvert, close acquaintance will bring to light the curious contrast between inner assurance and a hesitating and somewhat suspicious attitude towards the outer world.

A person of the *extravert thinking type* directs his life according to the facts of the outer world, and to the principles of the community in which he lives. This type is most often found among men. It will make a great difference whether, in addition to their thinking function, persons of this type make most use of Sensation or of Intuition, that is to say, whether their Thinking is chiefly occupied with sorting perceptions or impulses. In the first case, their Thinking will be of a businesslike character. Among the scientific men of our day we find many instances of the valuable work performed by this function in discovering and grouping new facts. But if it is Intuition that comes second in importance, Thinking will occupy itself more with sorting the potential ideas and motives of conduct which are or have been current in the life of the community. We find an instance in those philosophers whose work is chiefly concerned with the history of philosophy, and with co-ordinating the views of various thinkers, a process in which creative work may to some extent be achieved.

If the thinking function is of a less remarkable quality, and lacks such creative power, the disadvantage of its being the predominant function will be more apparent. The businesslike quality may often degenerate into dry dullness: the generally accepted principles and systems may become mere strait-jackets, and so be a hindrance to many valuable possibilities of development. The feelings especially will be repressed, so that expression will lack all liveliness and individuality. Nor will expression occur immediately; for the first impulse or reaction is held back until it has been tested by the systematised experience. Good and evil, right and wrong are judged according to whether they fit into this system, which has an absolute validity in the eyes of the thinking type. For them it is the purest expression of the laws of the universe. This applies to their scientific systems as well as to their ethics. Whatever does not fit into them, they regard as untrue, or as an exceptional chance. They are convinced that after due consideration, such facts can be made to agree with their system; and if they find something in their own nature, which cannot be reconciled with their ethics, they regard it as a chance imperfection, which they are sure some day to get rid of. They are also ready to reject as abnormal or morbid everything that does not fit in with their ideas. Yet if their point of view is wide enough, such persons often have a purifying and co-ordinating influence on contemporary thought. But if they have a narrow personality, they are apt to become niggling cranks. Their activity is most fruitful in an outward direction, and when they are giving shape to new material. Their systematising will then produce new ideas and clearness of vision. But if, on the other hand, they find everything already fixed into a system, they will aim merely at maintaining the *status quo*, and resist every innovation in the most conservative manner. They often cause all spontaneity to dry up both in their own domestic circle and in their inner nature.

If they do not entirely suppress their feelings, they allow only a small amount to be expressed through carefully regulated channels and according to definite principles. As these principles depend a great deal upon the outer world, it is evident that their emotions will often appear very conventional. But sometimes suppressed feelings may suddenly and unexpectedly arise out of the unconscious, and their expression will then seem quite inconsistent with conventional principles and emotions. Such inconsistency will appear in a sudden fit of violent temper, or in a case where altruism, founded upon principles, is perverted or destroyed by selfish motives. It may also happen that they are driven by their feelings to use means to attain their object which are not in accordance with their principles. There is yet another inconsistency between their involuntary feelings and their conscious attitude. This conscious attitude is more or less impersonal, and sets aside personal interests if they clash with propriety and convention; whereas the unconscious feelings are very sensitive on the personal side, and if they find that someone does not agree with them, they are apt to be annoyed, and this annoyance may sometimes take the form of exaggerated sensitiveness, or be expressed by involuntary insults. Thus scientific discussions may easily become unnecessarily heated. In daily life too, we often see that quarrels about matters of principle give rise to antipathy. Though the thinking extravert lacks the conscious desire of the feeling type to bring together all shades of opinion into one harmonious whole, this desire may all the same be active in his unconscious mind. He will then feel compelled to group together a variety of experiences and co-ordinate them into one theory or principle, which he will apply and defend on all occasions with the enthusiasm of a fanatic. Instances of this are the Darwinian, who because of his improved version of the story of the Creation, considers that there is no value whatever in the Bible, and the enthusiastic Freudian, who when he has realised the powerful influence of infantile sexuality, relates all, or nearly all, later psychic activity to this early influence. They both fall victims to their tendency to stretch too far a theory which is only valid up to a certain point.

The activities of thinking extraverts are directed towards the outer world, from which they receive their chief impulses and motives. But their contact with others is not so extensive and intimate as in the case of the extravert feeling type. The systematised experience by which they test everything, interferes with their relations with the world, and so they give the impression of being cold and impersonal. Their facial expression will at once reveal this to anyone of the feeling type. Their emotional relationships often present difficulties, because conventional expressions prove inadequate, and unconscious feelings may cause disturbances. Yet these thinking extraverts are usually well adapted to their surroundings, especially in practical matters. Here they are continually stimulated by their environment, and owing to their adaptability they are usually successful in their activities, which are often regular and on a large scale. Thought, because it hinders impulsive actions, is an obstacle to the development of great energy. But on the other hand thinkers usually have their will-power well developed. I agree with Jung that the will is the expression of the consciously organised desires, although, especially in the intuitive type, energy may arise from an unconscious impulse, independently of will-power.

Thought also tends to make activity of a permanent character, so that persons of this type usually possess great persistence. They are particularly suited to scientific investigation, and to all the professions which demand in the first place a sense of order, accuracy and thoroughness. They are often better able to deal with material things than with human beings, for they are apt to be hampered by strait-laced opinions and forms of expression. As belonging to the thinking type, they lack the personal touch; and as extraverts, they lack understanding of the subjective side. As we have already said, their unconscious feelings may sometimes have a disturbing influence, which may give rise to morbid symptoms, such as doubt, suspicion and fear. In this case too the treatment required for restoring a better balance will consist in drawing the unconscious emotions into the consciousness and developing them.

People of the *introvert thinking* type are also guided by their systematised experience; but in their case it is chiefly the experience of their inner life. Their system is based upon facts collected by introspection, rather than by the senses, and is built up out of impressions and impulses. Although their system is a product of their own creative thought, they also make use of the thoughts and ideas of others, if they are suitable. They use their sensuous experiences as a test for their opinions; but these experiences have not such a decisive influence as with the extravert thinking type: they serve more as illustrations of laws which Thought has already been forced to accept on the ground of other experiences. Thus the disadvantage, as compared with the extravert thinking type, is that the point of view of the thinking introvert is not so exclusively based on facts. Yet this disadvantage seems to be compensated by a more delicate power of abstract thought and a deeper introspective insight. Such persons have a great deal of self-knowledge. The moral principles according to which they sort and classify their impulses, are at the same time an attempt at balancing their contradictory intuitions; but they usually do not consider these principles to be general laws applicable to everyone. They assume that other people also are subject to some inner moral law; but they are not so ready as the thinking extravert to take an objective interest in its content.

Thinking introverts also are chiefly to be found among the male sex. We have seen that Thought tends in any case to interpose its system of sensations and reactions between the individual and his surroundings; and the thinking introvert will be at an even greater distance from the outer world than the thinking extravert. Originally Jung considered this type to be the true introvert type. Like all other introverts, they strike one, even in their youth, by a certain reserve. A child of an introvert type is apt to be shy, quiet and timid, as though it did not feel at home in the world. Chance expressions and unexpected original remarks will from time to time show that the child observes and reflects a great deal. Introverts in general present a very different appearance among strangers from what they do among intimates, but even among intimates only a small part of their inner life will be revealed. Thus thinking introverts will always most carefully consider and select their forms of expression. It is only under violent emotion that their reasoned self-control is broken through, and reactions appear which do not seem to fit in at all with their usual attitude of reserve. When they are pronouncing an opinion, they strike one as somewhat cold, obstinate and arbitrary. One feels as if they thought: "that is my opinion, which shall not be altered, whether you agree with it or not." No doubt they avoid conflict as much as possible, for every introvert intensely dislikes being forced to expose himself to the outside world; they will therefore maintain a certain distance by means of a stiff or polite attitude or even of apparent friendliness. But in most cases this attitude is not very convincing: it is easily felt to be a mask; and one is aware that they do not believe in it themselves, as thinking extraverts, for instance, believe in their conventional attitude. Thinking introverts are thus likely to be unsuccessful in their conventions (usually much to their regret, for they would be only too glad to mask themselves skilfully), and so their original emotions come to light sooner than in the case of the extravert thinking type. In their own small circle they may be looked upon as witty and original, though sometimes also as difficult and hot-tempered. Sometimes again a stiff and reserved person may show a very gentle and sensitive side to his immediate neighbours. Or else they may combine all these various qualities; for their emotional side is undeveloped, and contains a mass of unsolved contradictions. In questions of feeling, they are often very helpless and dependent upon others, and so are easily exploited.

Great freedom of growth and many delicate shades exist in the inner domain of their ideas and principles. But their special difficulty is that they do not know how or where to adapt their ideas to the world. They find it incomprehensible that what seems so clear to them is not always clear to others. So they take but little pains to express themselves lucidly. Jung writes about them (XXVI, p. 551): " Even if they get so far as to give their thoughts to the world, they do not deal with them as a careful mother does with her children, but expose them as foundlings, though they will be much annoyed if their ideas fail to make their way." A thinking extravert will be hampered in literary work by his wish to include in it the views of other writers by means of endless quotations and notes; whereas the thinking introvert will be held up by all kinds of reflections, limitations and additions, which make his progress slow and his work clumsy and unreadable. Kant is a good instance of the introvert, and Darwin of the extravert type.

The lack of assurance in persons of the introvert thinking type is shown by their attitude towards their surroundings and by their manners, which are often very awkward, being either exaggeratedly correct, or childishly negligent. Since all emotional problems present them with insoluble difficulties, they will avoid them if possible; but if they are unavoidable, they will try to find salvation either by clinging on principle to conventional forms, or else, equally on principle, by venting their feelings in undifferentiated forms of expression. Thus there is in reality a close connection between the idealists, who talk enthusiastically about pure love, and condemn and loathe all sexuality, and those who defend general lawlessness, because they think that no restraint should be put upon nature. A man of this kind, when he is in love, will always feel awkward, uncertain and ridiculous. He will try to escape from his difficulty of expression by attempting to persuade himself that it is merely a transient affection, or that the girl is not so attractive after all. If he does not succeed in this, he will try to express himself, and then it is often remarkable what exaggerated importance he attaches to minutiæ of expression. His emotions will urge him to hold forth at length about unimportant details, in order to persuade himself that the state of things is such as he would like it to be in reality. This tendency may also be present in the unconscious, when the emotions have been entirely repressed, and will then be sometimes revealed in an unpleasant manner. My experience with patients makes me think it probable that most of those suffering from persecution mania belong to this type.

Most thinking introverts are painfully conscious of their lack of adaptability, and this often causes them to feel inferior. They may hide this from the outer world by pride or apparent conceit ; but inwardly they will always feel themselves to be in the wrong. This sense of inferiority is also connected with the way they classify and organise their impulses. They build up an ideal about themselves, to which their desires and actions are meant to correspond. This happens with introverts of other kinds ; but in the case of the thinking introvert, his ideal is formed in accordance with his thought-system. As the feelings and desires which this system deals with, are not restrained by the natural limitations of reality, the ideal will often be affected and unnatural in character, and quite unlike what would be possible in reality. For the feeling introvert, such an ideal is a practical matter, in so far as he desires to see himself idealised in the opinions of other people whose judgment he respects, or wishes to imitate someone who embodies this ideal for him. But the ideal of the thinking introvert is far more a product of his fantasy. The further it is removed from reality, the more will he feel himself to be inferior. Such an ideal may be connected with ambitions or erotic fantasies, which have almost no basis; and the fact that, although they cannot be realised, they yet provide a large amount of facile satisfaction, may sometimes create a deep and dangerous chasm between his real and his phantasy life.

I will use as an illustration the dream of a patient who began to grow conscious of this condition during treatment. He had been absorbed for a long time in ambitious fantasies, in one of which he figured as a general. He now dreamt that he was in command of a besieged fortress. First of all he saw the outside of the castle, and was struck by its curious shape. Its foundations sloped inwards towards the bottom, so that it seemed as if it rested on a relatively small base. He immediately reflected that the fortress would be difficult to defend, as that point might be easily sawn through. After that he found himself inside the castle, which then appeared to be a house in which he had formerly lived. He was walking round, dressed as a knight and holding a sword in his hand, giving orders to retreat into one part of the fortress, as it could not be defended any longer. He was going along a passage, when suddenly he found himself in one of the main streets of Amsterdam, and felt somewhat awkward to be walking among ordinary people dressed as a knight with a naked sword in his hand. At first he could not at all understand the meaning of this dream; and yet there may be found in it a remarkably plastic image of his mental condition. The castle which is built on too small a foundation and is therefore indefensible, represents the world of his ambitious fantasies, which the treatment was dealing with. And when he becomes aware of the impossibility of realising these fantasies, he sees himself in the ordinary world, dressed up as if for the stage, with a sword in his hand, which even in the dream strikes him as strange and ridiculous.

The plasticity of such a dream seems almost too obvious to be probable, and is a rare occurrence. It shows clearly the tendency of the introvert to withdraw from life into a fortified position. If this tendency is not so strongly marked, it may lead him to think out all his plans beforehand in the greatest detail, so as to be prepared for every eventuality. The thinking introvert who has been able to overcome his weakness and fear of action, may develop into an energetic and enterprising leader, who is not easily turned aside from his purpose. But if the type is markedly narrow, then he is in some danger of losing himself in theories which recede further and further from the facts of life, and of seeking satisfaction for his emotional needs in fantasies. Contact with other people may help to restore the balance.

The *extravert intuitive* type is more difficult to describe than the feeling or thinking types, because one of its chief characteristics is its instability and its great power of adapting itself. The unconscious mental processes of persons of this type make them aware of special possibilities, which will then influence all their actions, feelings and thoughts. Peaceful, well-balanced relations with their surroundings give them a sense of discomfort. They express themselves more immediately than the other types both in actions and in words, without taking thought beforehand, and without necessarily expressing much of their personality. They are always striving to realise the fulness of life by realising their own being in its various manifestations. At one moment they will attach enormous importance to certain human beings or problems, which will be forgotten or thrust aside as soon as they have served their purpose. Jung writes (XXXVI, p. 528) : "They give the impression, which they seem to share themselves, that they have just reached the most definite crisis in their lives, and that henceforward they will be incapable of acting or thinking in any different way. . . . And yet the day will come when this same condition, which now appears to them as a deliverance, will seem to them to be a prison, and they will feel compelled to act accordingly, notwithstanding all possible arguments to the contrary, and although it would be much more reasonable and practical not to upset the balance."

These intuitive people are apt to have lively, keen minds, and to express themselves easily and abundantly. They are less in contact with their fellow-beings than the extravert feeling type, because they are less able to elaborate their expression, and adapt it to others. They have also less inner unity than the thinking types, and their various forms of expression are less co-ordinated. They only consider others to be of importance in so far as they can assist or prevent the realisation of their own potentialities of development, as revealed to them by intuition ; and they are apt to judge thoughts and principles, and the ethical significance of their impulses, according to this one practical point of view, and not according to generally accepted standards. The only law which they recognise is the inner power which is urging them forward. Persons of a different type are often astonished at the assurance of the intuitions by which they are guided; but if their self-confidence forsakes them for a moment, they are completely at a loss. This dependence upon impulses is apt to make them somewhat fickle. A dream of a markedly intuitive patient gave me an interesting instance of this. He saw in his dream a large motor-lorry, which had just broken down, and he heard the bystanders protesting loudly against the wild way the chauffeur had been driving He defended him on the ground that such chauffeurs were constantly obliged to drive different cars, so that they never had a chance of growing familiar with one type of machine. The analysis showed that this dream symbolised an apology for his own mistakes caused by impetuosity. He had great difficulty in controlling himself, as he was continually being swayed by new impulses and emotions.

Such intuitive persons are often very active, because they involuntarily tend to apply all their energy to whatever may arise at the moment; but they are usually impatient for results, and have a great need of variety. They display more impulsive energy than concentrated will-power. They are especially at home in those circumstances, where quick decision and ready action are required, as in business, in surgery, or in difficult military operations: but they often lack the capacity to carry on the work systematically, and bring it to a successful conclusion. This type is probably found as often among women as among men;

but women tend to use their intuition more in social life, and for the purpose of attaining some definite object If their personality is not too narrow, intuitive extraverts may be of great use in the world as discoverers and propagators of new ideas. Their judgments are founded on immediate conviction, rather than on elaborate thought ; and they often provide a ready solution to some problem, while reason lags behind, entangled in long arguments. Of course their intuition may sometimes be wrong, and then they will make profound mistakes, because they have no means of controlling themselves. But if they become aware of their mistakes, they usually know how to hide or disguise them with great skill. The difficulties that other people have to struggle with, seem to leave them unaffected, for they are extremely clever at escaping from tight corners. In spite of their usual spontaneity and cheerful energy, they are subject to moods of depression and uncertainty, which they will always try to hide as much as possible.

Intuition strongly influences both feelings and thoughts in this type, with the result that they are lively and often original, yet at the same time self-centred. They express their feelings even more than the feeling type ; and though the form of their expression is less elaborated, it is always spontaneous and often very original. Many wits and artists belong to this type. Their feelings are rarely permanent, and they do not feel the need of arousing similar feelings in others. They only seek to satisfy their own need of expression. It therefore often happens that such people can carry on long conversations without paying any attention to the answers and remarks of the person they are talking to. When they try to arouse a reaction in other people, it is only with a special object, and not because they wish to get into closer contact with them. Indeed they rather fight shy of this, as they are anxious not to lose their freedom of intuitive action. They frequently have a great number of acquaintances and friendly relations with people, but no really intimate friends. Their contact with others is very restricted, and as though limited almost to a single point; but as this is a very mobile point, it seems much greater than it is, and its mobility prevents adhesion or intimacy. This tendency to keep people at a distance depends upon a hardly conscious inner feeling of uncertainty, which is disguised by their apparent decisiveness. As long as they can deal with immediate events, their intuition will give them assurance; but when they have to meet the assurance of others, especially if it is based on sound arguments and fully developed thoughts and feelings, the implied criticism of their own assurance is so painful to them that they try to avoid it. They usually dislike defining their thoughts or feelings too precisely, because this would deprive them of spontaneity, which they value above everything else.

We must regard their ego-centric quality rather as a peculiar psychic form of reaction, than as an expression of egoism. Both Thinking and Feeling aim at the discovery of some common human ground as a basis for adaptation. With the feeling type, this basis will be found in the elaborated feelings that are common to everyone: with the thinking type it will consist in some common system of thought: while in the intuitive type adaptation will be based upon the individual expression of the instincts. Now surrounding influences may very easily confuse and disturb this expression, so it is an absolute necessity to the intuitive extravert not to allow these influences to affect him too much. Of course, there may be real egoists among this type: but they are also found among the feeling and thinking types; and it is just as likely that impulsive actions may be under the influence of non-egoistic intuitions. All the same we may assume that the development of the feeling and thinking type, especially of extraverts, usually leads away from the self towards more common human ground, while the development of the extravert intuitive type is ego-centric and aims rather at the realisation of the self. Therefore the danger of egoism is greater with them than with other extraverts, and it will chiefly depend upon the nature of their aims whether their expressions are of value to the community, or only to themselves.

There are fewer conflicts in the emotional life of the intuitive than of the feeling type. It is true their feelings are more full of contradictions; but these do not have such a disturbing effect, because the feelings are less developed, and contact with the outer world is more mobile and varied. Their ego-centric tendency is shown by the fact that usually they only display enthusiasm for a cause when they are able to play an important part in it themselves; and the rare occasions when they show enthusiasm for other people depend upon the amount of appreciation which they receive from them. A person of the feeling type is equally sensitive to the opinions of others about himself; but his reaction is more elaborated: he will weigh the criticism very seriously and may even worry for days about some unpleasant critical remark; whereas the intuitive type will show his childish vanity by trying to avoid any criticism, or by assuming a hostile attitude towards it.

In intellectual matters, persons of the intuitive type show the same lively originality, combined with an egocentric tendency. They can argue with great intelligence and are often considered authorities on various questions. They use their thought exclusively in order to obtain some definite result, never as an end in itself, as with the thinking type. At school, these types are often the despair of their teachers, because though obviously intelligent, they refuse to exert and develop their mental powers, unless they clearly see some immediate advantage in doing so. Since they do not rely upon Thought as the most important function, they often do without it, and the result is that their knowledge is often somewhat fragmentary and their theories may be quite illogical. Thus intellectually they resemble the feeling type; yet they may be of value to science, because their mental energy will lead to discussion and research. In matters of the intellect as well as of feeling, the intuitive will avoid being too closely bound by fixed formulas and laws, and he will try to avoid joining any special party, either in science or in politics. He seldom expresses his thoughts in a very definite form, and always seems to keep some of them in reserve. This may give an impression of insincerity or even of dishonesty; but the true reason is his desire for freedom of intuition. The many-sidedness and versatility of intuitive extraverts will often make them excellent go-betweens. But in spite of their apparent freedom of mind, they are often bound by conventional opinions and ideas borrowed from other people, and thus satisfy their need to find a counterpoise to their own instability. The great variety and fruitfulness of an intuitive extravert may be so exaggerated as to lead to sterility. Other persons who are patient and persistent enough to work out his ideas, may then reap the benefit of them, and the superficiality of the originator's mind will thus become evident. In such a case peculiar reactions from the unconscious may come to the surface in the form of pathological symptoms, the effect of which is to prevent him from living intuitively. It is evident that the treatment here necessary should aim at developing the compensating functions.

Introvert Intuition values inspiration above everything else, because it opens the way to new possibilities of development, which may not have much practical value, yet may be of great artistic, moral or religious value to humanity. The significance of such inspiration is often at first difficult to understand, because it is so vaguely expressed. This type includes mystical dreamers, prophets, and persons of fantastic imagination. William Blake seems to me a good example of an artist of this type. When such persons are not able to express their originality in art, they appear to be "possessed." As Jung says, they are suitable characters for psychological novels. They are always discovering in themselves wonderful thoughts and feelings, images and impulses, to which they often sacrifice their outward adaptation, and so may become extremely wayward in their behaviour. If they attempt to turn their intuition onto moral problems, they will aim at making their own life a realisation of their intuitive point of view, and will tend to find symbolic meanings in everything. As prophets they do not meet with much recognition, since their expression is so little adapted to their surroundings. Though their beautiful, somewhat vague theories and visions seem to lift them above ordinary human beings, yet, to the critical observer, they often appear to be unconsciously bound by various material concerns. This, according to Jung, is the compensating extravert sensation function, which, in its unconscious and undeveloped state, binds them to simple, instinctive impulses and sensations. If too little attention is paid to this compensating tendency, neurosis may result.

Persons of the *extravert sensation* type are governed by their impressions, to which they react under the influence of their instinctive desires. Facts, as perceived by the senses, are to them the only reality. They do not concern themselves with speculation or principles: they are realists to an extreme degree. They do not feel the need of formulating their experiences into a system, but their reactions are continually urging them forward from one sensation to another. Their attitude is not entirely passive, for they show a certain degree of psychic activity in the way they are affected by external impressions. But this activity is chiefly unconscious, and much less marked than in the intuitive type. It would not be true to say that they are entirely without principle, or that their life is unrestrained. Sensual pleasure is their chief object in life; but they require restraint, discipline, and a certain amount of self-sacrifice and public spirit in order to get the most out of life, just as much as do the other types when developing their special functions to the highest degree. Thus their life is not without order, which is based, not on personal principles or feelings, but on traditions and customs, upon which humanity has relied throughout the ages. We must be careful not to underestimate the importance of such tradition, since the whole organisation and stability of human society depends upon it. Persons of the extravert sensation type, more than any others, will find how dangerous it is to forsake the old paths which have stood the test of time.

A great many so-called ordinary people belong to this class. Their only striking quality may be that they are masters in the art of living. They are pleasant people, good comrades and gay companions. They often have great powers of observation, and so make excellent doctors and engineers. Their tendency to collect and classify large numbers of facts, is akin to the love they sometimes show of collecting objects of æsthetic or scientific interest. Persons with good taste and an æsthetic appreciation of the higher pleasures in life, belong to this type, although they would often regard themselves as belonging to the feeling type because of their great sensitiveness. They are often clever at arguing about the problems and theories of life, but they do so more for the sake of conversation than of the problems themselves. In order to experience certain sensations, they will launch forth into all kinds of subjects to which they are usually quite indifferent. They seek strong and special sensations, not merely pleasant ones. They try to bring the outward appearance of their life into harmony with their ideals. They dress well, live in comfortable surroundings, and have good manners and the necessary variety in their conversation and way of living. They often have a great knowledge and love of nature, but are very little concerned with the inner side of their life. Any expression of this inner life which might upset their happiness, is thrust aside as morbid. They are apt to make the mistake of considering the feelings and thoughts of others as akin to their own sensations. Their activity chiefly lies in reacting, and in making the necessary effort in order to obtain their sensations.

In some cases, such as coarse, sensual natures, or selfish æsthetes, the search for sensations is very strained. The other functions will then appear as the expressions of the unconscious: but I have no space here fully to describe the nature of such phenomena, because I should then have to deal at some length with primitive psychology and pathological questions. The treatment of persons of this type is always very difficult, as they do not find it easy to get to know themselves, or to develop their undeveloped functions into useful mental instruments. They often obstinately persist in ascribing their symptoms solely to physical causes, and find great support for this view in contemporary medical science.

Persons of the *introvert sensation* type are governed by their inner sensations, and like the other types that are governed by irrational or empirical functions, they are dependent upon the chance event. What is important to them is not the cause or objective strength of any given sensation, but the degree of their susceptibility to it, which might be called the subjective side of sensation. Such sensitiveness to sensation may on occasions predominate in everyone; but in this type it is the outcome of the inherited disposition and early experiences combined, and so predominates over all other functions, and the whole mental life is adapted to it. If outward circumstances have no disturbing influence, this adaptation may satisfy all inner needs. As in most cases this inner satisfaction does not reveal itself to the outer world, such persons often appear to be very unhappy and will receive much undeserved sympathy. They usually give the impression of being reserved, quiet and passive. The special quality of their sensations only appears in exceptional cases, for instance if they are artists: otherwise any original characteristics they may possess will remain almost completely hidden, though the outsider may be vaguely aware that there is something remarkable about them. This habit of keeping their inner life entirely to themselves without taking any pains to express it, may be attractive to some people, but is likely to be irritating to most.

Persons of this type generally suppress the spontaneous and impulsive side of their nature, because it would interfere with their receptivity. As their reserve prevents them from receiving much outside stimulus, they are not usually very active. Their lives lack a conscious direction and they have little concentration of will-power. Their outward circumstances are often out of harmony with their desires, and they may react to this in two different ways.

a. They may try to adapt themselves to the claims of the outer world, and will tend to regard their own sensations as morbid when they differ from those of others. Consequently they will suffer from a sense of inferiority.

b. They may turn away still further from the outer world, and withdraw entirely into themselves. Any adaptation to others will seem to them mere hypocrisy; and they sometimes show great cleverness in belittling other people's motives and ideals. All this is an inferior outlet for repressed intuition; and when such intuition becomes obsessive, a more serious conflict will arise. The lack of inner satisfaction will then cause a state of apathy and depression, with occasional unexpected intuitive outbursts in the form of over-excitement or aggressiveness.

It is of great importance that such persons should counteract their passiveness and dependence upon chance events by regular work and discipline; also that Thinking and Feeling should help them to find some sort of contact with the rest of the world. They will then gradually discover new and valuable forms of self-expression, and they will avoid the disturbing influence of their unconscious impulses.

To conclude this résumé, I will call attention to a few points which I have not yet dealt with. It should be understood that there are no clear lines of demarcation between these types. They are all developed out of a more primitive type of man, in whom these functions, guided by instinctive needs, co-operated in a more unconscious way. Any onesidedness in the development of these functions will in the long run give rise to some compensation ; and if this way of development is understood and followed, the various divergent types will be gradually brought nearer to each other. One function rarely predominates to such an extreme degree as to exclude all others ; as a rule other functions are used as well, so that there is a continuous gradation from one type to another. Accordingly this classification, like all classifications of character, may well appear to be somewhat arbitrary. Jung himself does not deny that other methods of classification are possible, or that other fundamental functions might be discovered. Nevertheless it seems to me that Jung's method of differentiating the types by means of their various forms of adaptation is one of his most fruitful ideas, and that the way he applies it to his practical work is as important as the insight which Freud has given us into the origin of various psychic products.

Jung's book on this subject deals with many points which I have only been able to treat in a summary way. It includes a comparison between other methods of classification and his own, showing that they are often very similar, though they do not cover so much ground. He also gives numerous details of the history of humanity, dealing with them from the point of view of contrasted types, and tracing various efforts that have been made to solve these contrasts. He proposes to deal in a future volume with the technique of his treatment. Jung's theory about types is only the beginning of the work that will have to be done upon this subject, and a vast amount of material will have to be tested and worked over, before we can attain to any scientific certainty. Freud and his followers have been able to collect a larger amount of material in support of their theories than Jung has yet done for his; and more time is required before their validity can be finally tested.

I cannot agree with the opinion of many of Freud's followers that Jung's theories are superficial and unimportant as compared with Psycho-analysis proper, or that he has contributed very little that is of value. The followers of Freud, thrilled by the new possibilities of understanding their patients, which their discovery of the unconscious has given them, have directed their minds chiefly to that side of psychology, and emphasised the contrast between the conscious and the unconscious. It seems to me that Jung has made an important advance by drawing attention to the possibilities of co-operation between the conscious and the unconscious, and by maintaining that the conscious psyche is the organised and sublimated part of the mind. In my opinion this in no way detracts from the genius of Freud, but it makes psychology a more complicated and difficult subject.

Freud's teaching has given us information about certain characteristic disturbances and difficulties; while in addition we have learnt from Jung the solution of these difficulties, and the various typical possibilities of development. Whereas Freud's psychology shows us clearly the faults and failures of others, Jung's theory of types helps us to appreciate their different ways of adaptation, and to understand their success. It will also throw light on the contrasts and misunderstandings between the types, which are such frequent obstacles to co-operation and sympathy among human beings. I will now give a short description of these contrasts.

It would seem that the widest contrast is that between extreme cases of extravert and introvert. The extravert impresses the introvert as superficial and satisfied with mere appearances. The introvert finds it difficult to distinguish between his own conventional adaptation and the extravert's personal adaptation. On the other hand, the extravert looks upon the introvert as a self-satisfied, eccentric and incalculable human being, because he believes him to be entirely dominated by the same strange impulses which he himself has experienced on rare occasions.

The difference between rational and empirical persons is no less marked. Any event can be regarded either as dependent upon law or upon chance; that is to say we regard it as dependent upon law if it fits in with our systematised thoughts or feelings, and upon chance if it does not do so. In so far as an event depends upon law, reason can deal with it. The empirical types do not rely on these systems; at any rate they do so much less than the rational types; and thus it is that they accept the element of chance much more readily than the thinking and feeling types. They are not so much irrational as empirical. Their rational side is a secondary function, and their dependence upon chance events makes them seem to the rational types to be opportunists and deficient in character. Conversely, the empirical mind finds it very difficult to conceive that anyone can value rational principles and ideals above the realities of life. If he imagines at all what they are like, he looks upon them as unpractical or theoretical fanatics, who would be more suitable for the profession of clergymen or university dons than for ordinary practical life.

The contrast between the thinking and feeling types is again quite different. Here too we see that one individual can judge another only by comparing him with himself. The result will be that a narrow thinking type will consider the feelings of the opposite type to be just as undeveloped, inferior and conventional as his own; while the feeling type will not take into account the thoughts and principles of the thinking type, because he expects them to be of as little value as he feels his own to be. Again, from the point of view of the thinking type with its fixed laws, the feeling type will seem to be as variable and fickle as the sensational or the intuitive type. But to the feeling type, the thinking type will appear to be always making use of circumstances in a cold, hard and calculating manner. This is somewhat the same impression as is produced upon him by the businesslike adaptation of the intuitive or the sensation type.

The sensation and the intuitive types are also opposed. The quiet adaptation to facts and to emotional needs, and the desire not to depart from historical tradition, which characterise the sensation type are very different from the active, restless search for possibilities and change which we find in the intuitive type. Here again each type will judge the predominating function of the other by comparing it to his own undeveloped function. The intuitions of the sensation type disturb the enjoyment he is seeking; but if the contrast between his functions is not too great, these intuitions will provide him with agreeable and varied experiences. Thus he will regard the intuitive in one way as a fickle and restless being, who fails to enjoy life because of sudden impulses and fancies, while in another way he will look upon the originality of the intuitive as a valuable addition to the sensations to be got out of life. Again, the freedom of the intuitive is sometimes unpleasantly restricted by sensations arising from the unconscious, and he will infer that similar restrictions exist in the sensation type, although the latter may give an impression of calm assurance.

All these contrasts may be still further complicated in various ways. Thus a thinking introvert will find it very difficult to understand a feeling extravert, and in a different way he will feel at a loss with an intuitive or sensational extravert. When we consider all these opportunities for misunderstanding, we may well wonder that human beings have all the same discovered so many useful forms of contact. But in the first place we must remember that such misunderstandings are the cause not only of unjustified contempt and repulsion, but also of unexpected appreciation and attraction. Thus it may happen that someone, who is aware of his own shortcomings, may for that very reason appreciate in others the special adaptations which he himself lacks. This appreciation is sometimes exaggerated at moments of psychic crisis. Introverts in particular often suffer from such exaggeration: and this gives them a sense of inferiority. Conscious agreement in their judgments may cause an involuntary bond between the thinking and feeling types, just as a common experience of chance events may be a bond between the empirical types. But such relations may also be due to unconscious causes. We often find that strongly opposed types, who do not in the least understand each other, nevertheless attract one another as if by magic. We can partly explain this by the fact that for practical purposes they complete each other, as often happens in marriage or in business associations. But this does not explain the process by which they discovered one another. Moreover these relations often exist without any practical object or result. We must therefore assume that some unconscious undeveloped function is urging one of them to discover in the other that more developed form of the same function, of which he is in such need for his own development. Although in some cases part of this process may be conscious, yet such relations do not really admit of a conscious examination, for then the contrasts would be brought to light and would cause mutual disparagement, because what is of most value in one mind is just what is inferior in the other.

This attraction between contrasted types is certainly not the only, nor the chief bond in which the unconscious plays an important part The undeveloped, unconscious function of one person may be attracted by a similar undeveloped but conscious function in another, as when a girl, who has been very strictly brought up, is fascinated by a libertine and rejects all parental advice, or as when an honest business man feels bound, against his better judgment, to place himself in the power of a man of bad reputation. Freud has given many illustrations of similar unconscious attractions in his psychological writings.

Thus we see that sympathy, as well as antipathy, may give rise to numerous misunderstandings. Hence there is great need of a psychology which may help us to understand the differences between the various types. Such a psychology should also throw light on the contrasts between nationalities. It is of course absurd to judge a whole nation as if it were a single individual ; yet we see that a nation will cling to certain definite ideals, which are those of its average individual, and will impose them through the medium of education. Hence the culture of one nationality often shows the characteristics of a special type. It is much easier to explain the contrast between French and German mentality, if we realise the importance of Feeling to the Frenchman, and the predominance of Thinking in the German ; and a similar method should help us to understand the impulsive intuitive American, and the Englishman with his differentiated sensations and his respect for tradition.

CHAPTER VI

THE RELATION BETWEEN THE CONSCIOUS AND THE UNCONSCIOUS

INVESTIGATIONS into the unconscious processes have very largely modified and extended our conception of the unconscious mind. Formerly only certain strictly limited psychic processes were conceived of as unconscious, and it was thought that these could at times be made conscious, though not without difficulty. These unconscious processes suggested a hypothetical explanation of many mysterious symptoms. This view is held by Freud in regard to a great part of these processes. He also considers that extensive introspection, helped by the study of dreams and fantasies, can bring to light many unconscious processes. But besides these, he assumes the existence of active unconscious processes which cannot be made conscious, and whose existence can only be proved by observing their influence on the conscious mind. Here also the unconscious is the hypothetical explanation of various conscious disturbances; but it is more difficult to produce immediate proofs to support it. However such hypotheses are always allowed in science, on condition that they are continually being tested by facts. We find numerous instances in natural science (XVIII, p. 29) such as the theory of atoms and molecules, which no one has ever directly perceived, yet to which we ascribe powerful energies. We could extend this comparison by saying that just as all material events are based upon atoms and molecules, so all perceivable psychic events are based on unconscious psychic processes. Freud gradually reached this conclusion through the theory that instinctive desires are the basis of the entire psychic life. This theory has really carried him beyond psychology, the task of which consists in tracing the laws of the psychic life without troubling to discover upon what it is based. Freud is aware of this, and therefore talks of meta-psychological theories (XIV, p. 200) on the analogy of metaphysics, which aim at discovering the basis of physical phenomena. But in so far as certain *definite* unconscious processes are examined from the point of view of their relation to some consciously experienced result, this study should certainly form part of pure psychology.

Freud has drawn special attention to the fact that repression may be the cause why a desire, with all its related feelings and images, fails to rise into consciousness. Thus the unconscious would consist of the repressed or useless part of the mind. But this seems to me a somewhat narrow view, even according to Freud's own theories; for if we agree with him that conscious life is based on these unconscious forces, we should also admit the possibility that there may be some part of the unconscious which owing to various causes, quite apart from repression, has not been developed into consciousness.* Jung and Maeder have extended Freud's theories, by suggesting that this unconscious part of the mind is its undeveloped

* This would be called the "Primary Unconscious" according to Tansley (See Note, p. 113).

rather than its repressed side. They therefore look upon the unconscious as a source of development, instances of which we saw in dreams and in the inspirations of artists and inventors, as I described in a former chapter. We also saw that these expressions of the unconscious are sometimes the compensations of a one-sided development. We occasionally find entirely new material among these expressions, as in the remarkable experiences of telepathy and dreams, which the Society of Psychical Research has collected. Some forms of insanity also present us with quite new expressions of the unconscious. We often find delusions which cannot be traced back to the early life of the patients, and show a remarkable resemblance to the contents of the mind of primitive man. I may also mention the experiences of mystics, who hear voices or see visions when they are in a special state of mind. All these mental products depend upon the unconscious; and it is probable that, besides many regressive elements, they also contain some new creative elements.

It is difficult to base a comprehensive understanding of the unconscious upon the above theories alone. Freud's theory, which emphasises repression, seems unsatisfactory, because he does not sufficiently take into account the development of new possibilities out of unconscious impulses. Jung, on the other hand, regards the unconscious more as the inherited disposition, and he sees a remarkable connection between expressions of insanity, certain dreams, forms of art or scientific views on the one hand, and the forms of expression of our primitive ancestors on the other. He gives the name of "the collective unconscious" to that part of the mind which in the course of ages has been determined by the inherited form of brain-structure, and which we find expressed in the disposition common to all mankind. The various psychic products which we find in the history of human culture throughout the ages, such as ancient religions, mythologies and superstitions, often reveal striking similarities. These have convinced some scientists that the various ancient races must have had some means of contact, of which there is no record; but Jung ascribes the similarity to a common psychical structure of the unconscious mind. If we accept this theory, we shall find that these psychical products of the race are an excellent means by which to investigate the structure of the collective unconscious. The curious ideas which primitive man connects with natural phenomena, must then be regarded as the projected content of his own unconscious psyche. Freud and some of his pupils have also to some extent accepted this view (XVI), but they trace the origin of these psychic phenomena to the influence of environment, while Jung tries to discover in them a tentative and groping process of evolution Here again it seems to me that these two theories do not so much oppose as complete and correct one another.

The followers of both schools however agree that the various influences of the unconscious form a connecting link between the conscious life of modern man and the impulses, thoughts and feelings of another lower mental sphere, which bears some resemblance to the spiritual life of our primitive ancestors. But Freud, as we have seen, emphasises the importance of the experiences of early childhood in their influence upon development, whereas Jung tends to lay more stress on inherited disposition, which he explains by his theory of the collective unconscious.

Anyone who undertakes a serious study of the expressions of his unconscious psyche will experience a considerable extension of his conscious personality, since he will not only penetrate into earlier stages of his development and perceive the threads which bind his present life to his past, but he will also discover powers of a vague and remote nature which link him to the experiences and potentialities of his race. This extension of his inner experience is not without danger, because the conscious content of his mind is apt to grow vague and chaotic, and so may seriously threaten his organised spiritual life and lead to insanity. It is therefore desirable that the investigation of the unconscious should be made under the systematic guidance of an experienced doctor, in order that the newly discovered material may be immediately organised. It is most inadvisable to treat Psycho-analysis as an amusing game or pastime Self-analysis should only be undertaken by those who are aware of its serious character and of its dangers, and who are in real need of it. This may explain and justify the objections which many healthy people entertain against this stirring up of the unconscious. They usually feel completely remote from such things and are content to remain so.

So far, the synthetic method of introspection has been used to advantage chiefly in the case of patients who wished to get rid of disturbing symptoms. But it may very well prove that a general application of this method will be of great assistance to the development both of the normal man and of the human race in general. It is clear that persons who are not much troubled by symptoms arising from the unconscious, will derive more benefit from a synthetic than from an analytic treatment; their aim will be to collect material for their further development, rather than to get rid of troublesome mental products Hence a genuine Freudian psycho-analysis rarely finds in healthy people any urgent motive for penetrating into their repressed spheres. Even where there are slight morbid symptoms with no particularly disturbing results, there does not seem to be sufficient reason for the analytic method. But the synthetic method, which aims at discovering all possibilities of development, by means of the expression of the unconscious, resembles much more closely the conscious strivings of many human beings; and this resemblance will help to overcome the resistance, which may occur in the course of introspection. Thus synthetic analysis is in close connection with conscious self-knowledge. Freud would probably regard this method merely as the process of bringing the pre-conscious into full consciousness; but this seems to me too simple an explanation.

We must now consider a question which is occupying the minds of many psychologists of our day: what is the relative importance of conscious and of unconscious strivings in the development of the mind; and will a systematised investigation of the unconscious always lead to greater clearness and harmony in the individual's psychic development? We must first explain more exactly what we mean by psychic development. All living organisms develop through the interaction of outer circumstances and inner disposition, so that they are continually finding ever better adaptations to the demands of both. The growth of a tree adapts itself to the quality of the soil and the prevalent winds, while at the same time it realises more and more completely the inborn nature of the tree. Psychic development also contains these two aspects. The influence of the outer world is too evident to need explanation. Freud has increased our knowledge of it in many respects. But two opinions are possible as to the importance of the inborn disposition. We may either regard the conscious personality as being the genuine expression of the disposition, and attach little importance to the unconscious processes; or else we may consider that the inborn disposition is manifested chiefly in the unconscious processes, whereas the consciously organised part of the mind represents a more or less arbitrary expression of the disposition. Our opinion as to the value of introspection will depend upon which of these two views we hold.

If we turn our attention to the psychic event in ourselves, we find that this event is both complex and simple at the same time. For everything that we experience is experienced by our Ego, and is, as it were, assimilated by it. The fact that it is I, who have heard or seen, thought, felt or done something, creates a link between these various activities, and unifies them in our experience. When once we have become conscious of our Ego, we never again lose this consciousness; and yet we are never able to form a definite conception of our Ego. It is the power in us that thinks and acts and feels, and that comprehends the whole psychic activity (XXX, p. 225). We cannot perceive the Ego, any more than we can stand behind ourselves and watch our actions. We can come nearest to a conception of it in its aspect as a unity. It is a point without dimension; and if we were to attempt to extend this point, we should come to certain conditions or functions of the Ego, such as feelings or thoughts. But this is no longer the Ego; it is the Self or personality. The Ego is an entity enthroned above the Self, the contents of which it surveys. It is necessary to distinguish clearly between these two.

We seldom succeed in concentrating our attention upon the entity of our Ego, and we are just as seldom conscious of the fact that our present life is based on the whole of our past life, and that all our experiences may influence the present. This influence of the past usually works in our unconscious, and we are unconscious of the fact that past and present experiences become unified in our mind. We can however consciously differentiate between the two by means of introspection. If we turn our attention to the past, we shall see that our psychic life is much more complex than we had first thought; what seemed to us a simple impulse, then proves to be the product of an unconscious assimilation of a former experience. A feeling of sympathy can thus be explained as the result of old remembrances, which were called forth by a superficial likeness to someone we were fond of in our youth. The more conscious we become of this complicated process, the more clearly shall we perceive that all our experience constantly accompanies us and remains active. At the same time, we shall realise that we can never obtain a comprehensive view of those influences of the past in their entirety. This is partly the result of repression, as Freud has made clear, and partly because the complexity is too great for our consciousness to grasp it as a whole.

I should like to use, in a modified form, an image borrowed from Bergson (III, p. 165), and illustrate by a diagram the influence exerted on our psychic life by these two poles, the ego and the unconscious experience. He uses the image of a cone which contains the whole psychic event.

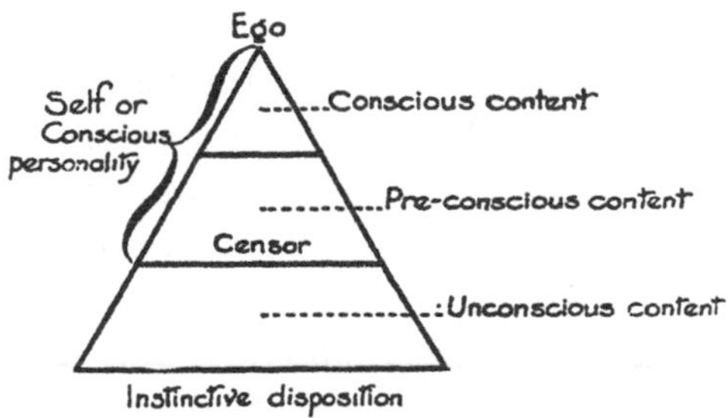

The apex represents the active Ego, while the basis contains the whole of the past experiences. Both poles together govern all psychic activity. If we also take into account Freud's theories, we must add that a part of this past experience is less immediately influential, because of the repressing activity of the censor. Under the influence of the conscious Ego, the constantly recurring contents of the mind are organised into selected groups of psychic experiences, which are of greater importance to us than any others. It is this organised Self that affects repression. This may explain what is meant by saying that "we were not quite ourselves." We mean that we went outside the narrow region which constitutes the Self, and our expressions were unlike those which we are accustomed to, and which are in harmony with our conscious organisation.

It is not my intention to go further into the philosophical side of these problems I only wished to point out that psychic events and qualities are not all related in the same degree to the conscious self or personality. The repressed unconscious processes are those that are furthest removed ; but other unconscious or preconscious processes can also be reckoned as belonging to the outer region of the Self. The interaction between the Ego and the preconscious and unconscious processes is quite constant and continuous. There is less interaction between the Ego and the repressed part ot the unconscious, but even there it is never entirely absent. The unconscious gives variety to the psychic event, the Ego gives stability and harmony to it. By bringing the unconscious part of the psychic event into consciousness, we shall discover the desires which underlie the psychic event, and be able to analyse the psyche into its various elements On the other hand a synthesis of the psyche may be arrived at by grouping together the various thoughts, feelings, sensations and intuitions under the control of the Ego. Consciousness is most intense where contradictions and difficulties are being solved by means of a unifying synthesis ; whereas one-sidedness, automatism and disconnectedness are characteristic of the unconscious. When unconscious desires and feelings are drawn into the consciousness, they tend to enrich and develop the psyche, while the activity of the conscious mind is directed towards grouping and organising its material.* Thus though the unconscious may be helpful in enriching and completing the mind, it is not suited to be the governing force because of its instability.

We have now arrived somewhat nearer to the answer to our question, which we can reformulate thus: which is of more importance to the development of the psyche, the organised unity provided by the consciousness, or the variety of possibilities arising from the unconscious? Evidently both are necessary to development, and we begin to perceive that their relative importance depends chiefly upon individual circumstances. Let us take as instances the extreme contrasts of A, whose mind is stiffened and stereotyped by his conscious principles, and B, who constantly lets himself go in answer to any chance sensation or inspiration. For A, the way to a new and richer life will be opened by raising to the conscious plane the unconscious, insufficiently organised side of his personality; while in B's case this same process would either increase the chaos or leave it untouched. A will quite naturally set about bringing the newly discovered facts into harmony with the rest of his personality; while this harmonising process is one which B will have to learn with an effort. The difference between A's point of view and B's, is much the same as the difference between Jung's rational and irrational types.

* In cases of psychic disturbance the unconscious is organised to a certain extent; and next to the nucleus of the personality we find what might be called a contranucleus. In obsessional neuroses this organisation is not very marked, but it appears clearly in cases of automatic writing or of dual personality in hysteria (p. 8-9), and it may also be observed in mediums or in the insane.

CHARACTER AND THE UNCONSCIOUS

In the last chapter I attempted to describe the various ways in which the conscious Self may develop, and its various relations to the unconscious; but this very variety made it difficult to explain what qualities these developing processes have in common. William James has treated this question extensively in his *Varieties of Religious Experience* (XX). He restricts the problem to a certain kind of change in the Self, namely to religious conversion; but this makes it all the easier to obtain a clear view of the matter, for religious development is closely connected with the general development of character. James describes conversion as a change in the nucleus of the personality, or as a new synthesis. He shows by a great many examples that this change may be brought about in a variety of ways. In cases of one kind, the process is chiefly conscious, though powerfully influenced by unconscious desires which are the cause of conflict and unrest. But there are other cases of an opposite kind, where the new nucleus arises and develops in the unconscious, so that the conversion takes place as a complete and sudden revolution. In such cases it would seem as though at the critical moment two beings were struggling to gain possession of the soul. This kind of conversion mostly occurs in people whose conscious mind is but little developed, and such striking regenerative changes often suggest the symbol of re-birth. If the change is more gradual, the conscious life will play a greater part in it, and it will merely appear to be a crisis in the psychic development. But in both cases the result will be a widening and unification of the personality. We have seen that this takes place in all psychic development; but the difference is that in a conversion, the contrast between the old and the new condition is much more marked than in a process which develops gradually. Sometimes, especially in intuitive persons, a less important change of the Self may suddenly arise out of the unconscious. But this kind of synthesis may simply be the revelation of a new undiscovered part of the disposition, and cannot be interpreted as a general reorganisation of the psyche.

In my opinion the word re-birth, if it is to be used at all in psychology, ought to be confined to those cases in which the new synthesis is a truer image of the disposition than the earlier one, and in which the nucleus of the Self has become more central after the change than it was before. It is only in those cases that the change will lead to a decrease of inner conflict, and an increase of strength and assurance, which will enable the individual to develop more in accordance with his inmost nature. We may illustrate this process by slightly altering our former diagram.

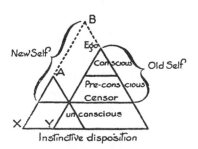

Some special circumstances in a person's life may sometimes awaken a new part (*x*-*y*) of the instinctive disposition. This may give rise to new unconscious processes, which may in part succeed in passing the censor, and may thus grow into a more or less independently organised group of psychic processes, which with its own apex A will be found in opposition to the conscious organisation. This will lead to an increasingly conscious solution, and to a more comprehensive standpoint of the Ego, which, from the apex B, will then embrace a new and wider organisation. It is evident that the extension of the organisation may be produced either by the growth of A or of the Ego.

Although this is only an incomplete description of the process of re-birth, it is sufficient to show the similarity between re-birth and the development at which psychological treatment aims Here also the relative importance of the part played by conscious and unconscious processes may be very different. One person will look upon his unconscious as the source of all creative power; while another, whose gradual development is governed by conscious tendencies, will look upon his conscious ideals as the guiding force in his life. Each of them mistakenly identifies his own method of obtaining unity and harmony with the resulting development itself, and this may give rise to considerable misunderstanding.

Psychic development can only be really understood by those who have first experienced it, and afterwards studied it introspectively. To them it appears as a process which is regulated by its own laws and principles, and which gives them an inner conviction and assurance Religious experience moreover gives rise to the conviction that this special form of development not only takes place in the individual, but is common to the whole of humanity as a creative principle. Thus the idea of religious re-birth will gain a metaphysical significance, in so far as it is held to imply a unification of ourselves with that deepest basis of our being which contains some of the cosmic energy operating in the universe outside the individual

Whatever may be the religious or metaphysical opinions of the psychological practitioner, he must be careful to distinguish them from his views on psychology, and psychological treatment, otherwise psychology will become the battlefield of beliefs of every kind, instead of a science based on experience, and the psychological basis of the unconscious will become confused with a metaphysical conception of the unconscious, such as von Hartmann considers to be the basis of all psychic and material events. According to that view the creative energy which is found in all vital processes, would only belong to the unconscious; whereas in point of fact it is also found in conscious processes and in organic life.

It may be useful to restate clearly what constitutes the similarity and the difference between a psychological treatment and a religious development. They are similar in so far as both deal with an inner conflict that arises when new regions and qualities of the psyche, opposed to the former unity of the conscious personality, begin to show themselves. In both cases the solution of this conflict is found in a new synthesis, which is at the same time a widening and a unification of the mind. In psychological treatment the success of the synthesis is measured by the patient's symptoms, which will reveal whether the inner conflict is solved. It is of secondary importance how far unity of organisation has been obtained, or the consciousness of an inner creative principle, which may lead to religious experience. But in a conversion or religious development, what is first aimed at is this consciousness of unity with the divine spirit; and this may subsequently lead to a solution of the inner conflict, and bring about a synthesis. Thus the ideal which is aimed at is very similar in both cases, but the road by which it is reached may be very different. As religions usually aim at a special kind of synthesis, it would be dangerous if psychology were to fall under their influence, for it might then lose some of its scientific objectivity. I hope that I have now shown that the latest psychology does not regard religion as a relic of primitive ages, which may be of historic interest, but can be of no use to a modern human being. Jung and Maeder especially have laid stress on the importance to mankind in general of this desire for harmony, both within the Self and in relation to the universe, which has been expressed by all religions throughout the ages; and with this opinion I am in complete agreement. It also seems to me that psychology can be of great help to us in deepening our understanding of religious processes, so long as it strictly confines itself to its own point of view.

We will now try to answer the practical question, whether systematic introspection leading to a discovery of the unconscious, is useful and desirable for the development of a human being. In the first place we must remember that the vital principle which organises the inner and outer experiences of the mind, does not work exclusively either in the conscious or in the unconscious. In most cases the development will proceed most satisfactorily when there is interaction between conscious and unconscious processes.

We shall usually find that in normal persons this interaction occurs naturally, without any special effort. The greatest men of all ages, when looking backwards on their lives, have often felt as though they had been urged forward in their development by some unknown power outside their own conscious will, and as though their surrender to this power had helped them more than any strained effort of will-power could have done. Thus it seems to me that a systematic hunting for products of the unconscious is by no means a necessity for development, and should certainly not be put forward as an ideal. In a normal development the necessary factors will naturally come forward when they are required

If we consider someone in a state of moral or religious conflict, we find that his attention is continually being drawn to certain thoughts and feelings arising from the unconscious, and that a conscious assimilation of these may help towards a solution. Although a similar predominance of products of the unconscious occurs in cases of mental illness, no unaided conscious assimilation is there possible; but psycho-analysis may bring a solution by providing insight into these unconscious processes by a method which only differs from the natural unaided solution of such conflicts by being more technical. In these morbid cases, a systematic assimilation of the products of the unconscious will help towards a solution, because in such mental disturbances the natural co-operation between the conscious and the unconscious is lacking.

It may also happen that the natural process of development has been disturbed, although there is no definite conflict between conscious and unconscious processes. The consciously organised mind may have grown so rigid that it is no longer capable of receiving new impulses and impressions. If in these cases we succeed in drawing the attention to the unconscious, the whole mental life may be intensified. This is also true of the life of the community, where the desire to escape from old rigid forms is shown by the appearance of various new forms of religion, art and politics, and also by a general interest in the more remarkable products of the unconscious. But where the development, both in the case of individuals and of communities, is not so much a natural growth arising from inner needs, as a conscious effort directed by the desire for development, there will be a danger that a condition of barbaric one-sidedness and discord will result. It therefore seems to me most important that, in spite of the excellent results of conscious treatment, we should never lose sight of the ideal development, which takes place according to its own natural laws and rhythm. A systematic method, which does not keep step with that inner rhythm, may do more harm than good. Freud has given excellent advice to practitioners on that subject, and has recommended certain precautions against arbitrary interference, which we should do well to follow in any treatment of the unconscious.

The increased understanding of the origin and solution of psychic conflicts will also be of special value to those persons who are consciously aiming at self-development, unaided by any treatment. By gaining insight into their problems, they will acquire the necessary patience and perseverance to allow the natural development to take its course, without disturbing it by strained efforts and experiments.

If a doctor is to guide a process of development, he must in the first place respect the law of development peculiar to his patient. He will only be capable of doing this, if he accepts and follows such a principle in his own life. Even then his task will be anything but easy, because this principle of development manifests itself in so many various ways, and because it is always extremely difficult to penetrate thoroughly into the psychology of others.

I venture to think that synthetic psychology will be of great help to human development in the future. It will lead to a greater respect for the freedom of individual growth, and it will also remove many sources of misunderstanding We shall come to realise that our conflicts about ideas and principles are often no more than disguised attempts to domineer and to suppress the opinions of others, who after all have as much right to their own ideas as we have. This point of view may shock those people who consider their own judgments to be the only right ones. But we hope that they may console themselves by the thought that the objective recognition of various possible theories will lead naturally to a new and more comprehensive point of view in psychology.

The future of this new psychology seems so vast and so full of possibilities, that it may well appear to some people as a mere speculative fantasy. In my opinion we are only at the beginning of this development, and it will require the efforts of many scientists through several generations to bring the work to perfection. In this book I have only been able to give the main outline of the new psychology, which attracts so many people who had sought in vain for help and enlightenment in the old academic psychology. Instead of looking upon the human mind as an engine, which we examine by taking it to pieces wheel by wheel, we now realise the unity of the psychic organism, and try to understand it in its coherent activity. In the course of this study we shall constantly meet with impenetrable mysteries, but the new psychology teaches us to recognise our shortcomings, and frankly to confess our ignorance. All our knowledge ends in realising that the basis of our life is mystery. A science which leads us to face this truth, brings us into contact with the deepest problems of our being.

BIBLIOGRAPHY

I. ALFR. ADLER, *Ueber den nervösen Character.* 1912.

II. W. F. HENRI BERGSON, *L'évolution créatrice.* 14e éd.

III. —— —— *Matière et mémoire.* 10e éd.

IV. E. BLEULER, *Affectivität, Suggestibilität, Paranoia.* 1906.

V. M. K. BRADBY, *Psycho-analysis and its place in life.* 1919.

VI. JOS. BREUER und Sigm. Freud, *Studien über Hysterie.* 2e Aufl.

VII. HANS DRIESCH, *Das Problem der Freiheit.* 2e Aufl.

VIII. SIGM. FREUD, *Zur Psychopathologie des Alltagslebens.* 3e Aufl.

IX. —— —— *Die Traumdeutung.* 3e Aufl.

X. —— —— *Sammlung kleiner Schriften zur Neurosenlehre.* 2e Folge.

XI. —— —— *Drei Abhandlungen zur Sexualtheorie.* 3e Aufl.

XII. —— —— *Formulierungen über die zwei Prinzipien des psychischen Geschehens. Jahrb. f. Ps. An. F.* B. 3. H. 1.

XIII. —— —— *Zur Einfuhrung des Narcismus. Jahrb. f. Ps. An. F.* B. 6.

XIV. —— —— *Das Unbewuszte. Intern. Zeitschr. F. Ps. An.* 3e Jahrg.

XV. —— —— *Vorlesungen zur Einführung in die Psychoanalyse.* 1916.

XVI. —— —— *Totem und Tabu.* 1913.

XVII. —— —— *Jenseits des Lustprinzips.* 2e Aufl.

XVIII. J. H. VAN DER HOOP, *Ueber die kausalen und verständlichen Zusammenhänge nach Jaspers. Zeitschr. f. d. ges. Neur. u. Ps.* B. 68.

XIX. HERMINE HUG HELLMUTH, *Vom "mittleren" Kinde. Imago.* B. 7. H. 1.

XX. WILLIAM JAMES, *The Varieties of Religious Experience.* 28th impr.

BIBLIOGRAPHY

XXI. PIERRE JANET, *L'état mental des hystériques*. 2e éd.

XXII. ERNEST JONES, *Papers on Psycho-Analysis*. 1918.

XXIII. C. G. JUNG, *Ueber Konflikte der kindlichen Seele*. 2e Aufl.

XXIV. —— *Wandlungen und Symbole der Libido*.

XXV. —— *Collected Papers on Analytical Psychology* (transl. C. E. Long).

XXVI. —— *Psychologische Typen*. 1921.

XXVII. ALPHONSE MAEDER, *Ueber das Traumproblem. Jahrb. f. Ps. An. F.* B. 5.

XXVIII. —— —— *Heilung und Entwicklung im Seelenleben*.

XXIX. MAURICE NICOLL, *Dream Psychology*. 1917.

XXX. KONSTANTIN OESTERREICH, *Die Phanomenologie des Ich*. 1910.

XXXI. HERBERT SILBERER, *Ueber die Symbolbildung Jahrb. f. Ps. An. F.* B. 3. H. 2.

XXXII. —— —— *Probleme der Mystik und ihrer Symbolik*. 1914.

XXXIII. A. G. TANSLEY, *The New Psychology and its Relation to Life*. 6th impr.

INDEX

INDEX

INDEX